Barre Workouts

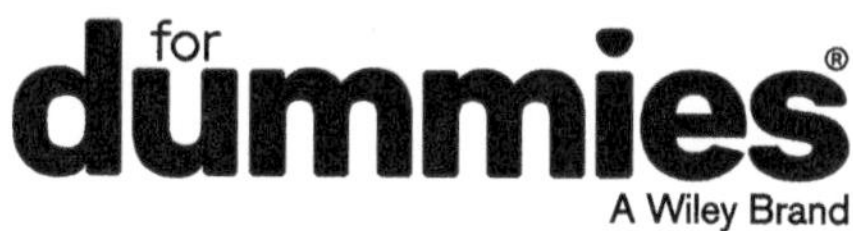

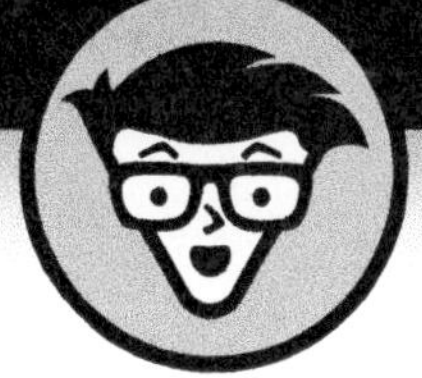

Barre Workouts

by Andrea Leigh Rogers

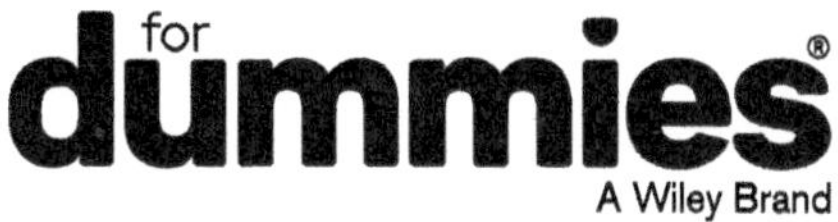

for dummies®
A Wiley Brand

Barre Workouts For Dummies®

Contents at a Glance

Introduction 1

Part 1: Getting Started with Barre Workouts 5
CHAPTER 1: Stepping Up to the Barre: A Barre Primer 7
CHAPTER 2: Reviewing the Barre Body 15
CHAPTER 3: Learning the Terms: Barre Talk 23
CHAPTER 4: Preparing for Your First Workout 33
CHAPTER 5: Getting into Position: The Main Moves 41

Part 2: Meet Me at the Barre: Component Exercises 73
CHAPTER 6: Warming Up 75
CHAPTER 7: Waking the Upper Body 89
CHAPTER 8: Barre Work Basics: The Classic Positions 123
CHAPTER 9: Strengthening Your Core 159
CHAPTER 10: Firing Up Your Lower Body 175
CHAPTER 11: Active Stretching 187

Part 3: Workouts That (Really) Work 207
CHAPTER 12: Full-Body Workouts 209
CHAPTER 13: Express Workouts 231
CHAPTER 14: Movement Snacks 245

Part 4: The Part of Tens 253
CHAPTER 15: Ten Important Barre Exercises 255
CHAPTER 16: Ten Ways to Supercharge Your Workout 261
CHAPTER 17: Ten Questions to Ask When Choosing a Class or Instructor 265

Index 271

Table of Contents

INTRODUCTION 1

    About This Book. 1

    Foolish Assumptions. 2

    Icons Used in This Book 3

    Beyond the Book 3

    Where to Go from Here 3

PART 1: GETTING STARTED WITH BARRE WORKOUTS 5

CHAPTER 1: **Stepping Up to the Barre: A Barre Primer** 7

    What Is a Barre Workout? 7

        Ballet-inspired exercise 8

        A series of small moves with big results 8

        Isometric holds 9

    Understanding the Fundamentals 10

        Strength 10

        Stamina. 10

        Stretch. 10

        Stability 11

    Why You Don't Need a Wall-Mounted Barre 11

    You Don't Have to Be a Dancer — In Fact, Far from It 11

    Practicing Barre for a Lifetime. 12

        Mind–body movement 12

        Sustainable strength and mobility 13

        Low impact, high intensity 13

        Natural stress reliever. 13

    Adding Modifications and Progressions 14

    Combining Barre with Other Forms of Exercise 14

CHAPTER 2: **Reviewing the Barre Body** 15

    Knowing Your Body from Top to Toe 15

    Head, Neck, and Spine 16

        Head 16

        Neck. 16

        Spine 17

    Shoulders and Arms 18

        Elevation and depression. 18

        Protraction and retraction 18

Core 18
    The "six pack" (yes, you probably have one!) 18
    Obliques 19
    Transverse abdominis 19
    Pelvis 19
    Butt 19
Knees, Ankles, and Feet 20
    Knees 20
    Ankles and feet 20
Muscle System 21

CHAPTER 3: **Learning the Terms: Barre Talk** 23
The Core: Your Power Center 23
    Pelvic control 24
    Posterior tilt 24
    Anterior tilt 24
    Neutral pelvis 26
    Navel to spine 26
    Creating a C-curve 27
Alignment and Posture: Building the Framework 27
    Neutral spine 27
    Neutral shoulders and arms 27
    Closed ribs 28
    Square off (or box) 28
    The midline 28
The Lower Body: Strength, Balance, and Power 28
    Foot stability and alignment 29
    Knee placement 29
    Isometric exercise 30
    Static stretch 31
Movement Mechanics: How You Move 31
    Lift with purpose 31
    Planes of movement 31
    Range of motion 31
    Supportive leg or arm 32
    Working leg or arm 32

CHAPTER 4: **Preparing for Your First Workout** 33
Setting Up Your Space 33
    Choosing the right equipment 34
    Wearing the right clothes 35
    Upgrading your experience with music 35

Examining the Main Components of a Barre Workout 36
    Warming up 36
    Starting with the upper body. 36
    Moving to barre (chair) work 37
    Strengthening your core. 37
    Focusing on floor work 37
    Cooling down and stretching. 38
Being Consistent 38
Staying Motivated 39
    Marking movements. 39
    Giving a full-out effort. 40
    Balancing mastery with novelty. 40

CHAPTER 5: **Getting into Position: The Main Moves** 41
Classical Ballet Positions. 41
    First position: Feet. 41
    First position: Arms 43
    Second position: Feet 44
    Second position: Arms 45
    Low fifth and high fifth positions: Arms. 46
    Port de bras 48
Technical Foundations 49
    Isolation 49
    Flexion. 50
    Extension 51
    Flexibility. 52
    Contraction. 54
Classical Movements. 54
    Plié. 55
    Tendu 56
    Relevé 57
    Passé. 59
    Développé. 61
    Devant, à la seconde, and derrière. 62
Classical Ballet Poses 63
    Attitude. 63
    Arabesque 65
    Penché. 66
Dynamic Movements and Training Concepts 67
    Battement. 68
    Pivot. 69
    Curtsy 70
    Challenge zone. 71

PART 2: MEET ME AT THE BARRE: COMPONENT EXERCISES 73

CHAPTER 6: **Warming Up** 75

Exercises in This Chapter 75

Knee-Lift Series 76

Getting set 76

The movement 76

Do's and don'ts 77

Variations 78

Plié Tendu 78

Getting set 78

The movement 79

Do's and don'ts 80

Variations 80

First-Position Lunge Back 81

Getting set 81

The movement 81

Do's and don'ts 82

Variations 83

Side Reach 83

Getting set 83

The movement 83

Do's and don'ts 85

Variations 85

Curtsy Pliés 86

Getting set 86

The movement 86

Do's and don'ts 87

Variations 87

CHAPTER 7: **Waking the Upper Body** 89

Exercises in This Chapter 89

Bicep Curl 90

Getting set 90

The movement 91

Do's and don'ts 94

Variations 94

90-Degree Lifts 94

Getting set 95

The movement 95

Do's and don'ts 97

Variations 97

Waltzing 97
    Getting set 98
    The movement. 98
    Do's and don'ts. 99
    Variations 100
Arm Circles 100
    Getting set 101
    The movement. 101
    Do's and don'ts. 103
    Variations 103
Port de Bras Arms 103
    Getting set 103
    The movement. 104
    Do's and don'ts. 104
    Variations 104
Hug and Carriage. 105
    Getting set 105
    The movement. 106
    Do's and don'ts. 108
    Variations 108
Swimming and Temperature. 108
    Getting set 108
    The movement. 109
    Do's and don'ts. 111
    Variations 111
V-Press 111
    Getting set 111
    The movement. 111
    Do's and don'ts. 113
    Variations 113
Rowing and Puppet. 113
    Getting set 113
    The movement. 113
    Do's and don'ts. 115
    Variations 115
Hinge Swing Fly Series 115
    Getting set 115
    The movement. 115
    Do's and don'ts. 116
    Variations 116
Curtsy Triceps 116
    Getting set 117
    The movement. 117
    Do's and don'ts. 118
    Variations 118

Triceps Lunges 119
    Getting set 119
    The movement. 120
    Do's and don'ts. 121
    Variations 121

CHAPTER 8: Barre Work Basics: The Classic Positions 123

Exercises in This Chapter 123
First-Position Pliés. 124
    Getting set 124
    The movement. 125
    Do's and don'ts. 127
    Variations 127
Second-Position Pliés 127
    Getting set 127
    The movement. 128
    Do's and don'ts. 129
    Variations 129
Fourth Position 129
    Getting set 130
    The movement. 130
    Do's and don'ts. 132
    Variations 132
Second-Position Cardio 132
    Getting set 132
    The movement. 132
    Do's and don'ts. 133
    Variations 134
Parallel Pliés 134
    Getting set 135
    The movement. 135
    Do's and don'ts. 137
    Variations 137
Hip Circles 137
    Getting set 138
    The movement. 138
    Do's and don'ts. 139
    Variations 139
Passé Press Series 140
    Getting set 140
    The movement. 140
    Do's and don'ts. 141
    Variations 141

Back to Barre Battements 142

    Getting set 142

    The movement. 143

    Do's and don'ts. 144

    Variations 145

Back Attitude 145

    Getting set 145

    The movement. 146

    Do's and don'ts. 146

    Variations 147

Ballet Lunges 147

    Getting set 147

    The movement. 147

    Do's and don'ts. 148

    Variations 148

Hamstring Series 148

    Getting set 148

    The movement. 149

    Do's and don'ts. 150

    Variations 150

Side Lifts 150

    Getting set 150

    The movement. 151

    Do's and don'ts. 152

    Variations 152

Resistance Band Series. 153

    Getting set 153

    The movement. 154

    Do's and don'ts. 154

    Variations 155

Fold-Over Series. 155

    Getting set 155

    The movement. 156

    Do's and don'ts. 157

    Variations 157

CHAPTER 9: **Strengthening Your Core**. 159

Exercises in This Chapter 159

C-Curve Hold 160

    Getting set 160

    The movement. 160

    Do's and don'ts. 161

    Variations 162

C-Curve Abs 162
        Getting set 162
        The movement. 162
        Do's and don'ts. 164
        Variations 165
Supine Lifts. 165
        Getting set 165
        The movement. 165
        Do's and don'ts. 167
        Variations 167
Scissors 167
        Getting set 167
        The movement. 168
        Do's and don'ts. 169
        Variations 170
Passé Abs 170
        Getting set 170
        The movement. 171
        Do's and don'ts. 171
        Variations 172
Planking 172
        Getting set 172
        The movement. 173
        Do's and don'ts. 174
        Variations 174

CHAPTER 10: **Firing Up Your Lower Body** 175
Exercises in This Chapter 175
Side-Seat Series 176
        Getting set 176
        The movement. 176
        Do's and don'ts. 179
        Variations 179
Love to Hate 180
        Getting set 180
        The movement. 180
        Do's and don'ts. 182
        Variations 182
Bottoms Up 182
        Getting set 182
        The movement. 183
        Do's and don'ts. 185
        Variations 185

CHAPTER 11: **Active Stretching** 187
  Stretches in This Chapter 187
  Upper-Body Stretch Series 188
    Getting set 188
    The movement 188
    Do's and don'ts 192
    Variations 192
  Seat Stretches 192
    Getting set 192
    The movement 192
    Do's and don'ts 194
    Variations 194
  Abs and Torso Stretch Series 194
    Getting set 195
    The movement 195
    Do's and don'ts 197
    Variations 197
  Full-Body Ballet Stretches 198
    Getting set 198
    The movement 198
    Do's and don'ts 199
    Variations 200
  Floor Stretches 200
    Getting set 200
    The movement 200
    Do's and don'ts 203
    Variations 203
  Balance Ending 204
    Getting set 204
    The movement 204
    Do's and don'ts 205
    Variations 206

PART 3: WORKOUTS THAT (REALLY) WORK 207

CHAPTER 12: **Full-Body Workouts** 209
  Full-Body 50-Minute Workout A 209
    What you need 210
    How to do it 210
    Warm-up 210
    Upper-body series 210
    Barre series 213
    Core series 215
    Lower-body floor series 216
    Stretches and balance ending 217

Full-Body 50-Minute Workout B 218

    What you need. 218

    How to do it 219

    Warm-up. 219

    Upper-body series. 220

    Barre series 220

    Core series 222

    Lower-body floor series 223

    Stretches and balance ending 223

Full-Body 50-Minute Workout C 223

    What you need. 224

    How to do it 224

    Warm-up. 224

    Upper-body series. 224

    Barre series 225

    Core series 226

    Lower-body floor series 226

    Stretches and balance ending 226

Full-Body 30-Minute Workout 227

    What you need. 227

    How to do it 227

    Warm up 227

    Upper-body series. 228

    Barre series 228

    Core series 229

    Stretches and balance ending 229

CHAPTER 13: **Express Workouts** 231

Express Upper-Body Workout. 231

    What you need. 232

    How to do it 232

    Warm-up. 232

    Upper-body sculpt. 232

    Optional cardio burst 233

    Balance 233

    Stretch. 233

Express Lower-Body Workout. 234

    What you need. 234

    How to do it 234

    Warm-up. 234

    Lower-body sculpt. 234

    Optional cardio burst 235

    Balance 235

    Stretch. 236

Express Core Workout 236
   What you need 236
   How to do it 237
   Warm-up 237
   Core series 237
   Optional core cardio 238
   Balance 238
   Stretch 238
Express Cardio Workout 239
   What you need 239
   How to do it 239
   Warm-up 239
   Cardio series 240
   Balance 240
   Stretch 240
Express Total-Body Workout 240
   What you need 241
   How to do it 241
   Warm-up 241
   Total-body sculpt 241
   Cardio burst 242
   Balance 242
   Stretch 242

CHAPTER 14: **Movement Snacks** 245
Snack-Sized Pliés 245
   Getting set 246
   The movement 246
   Do's and don'ts 246
   Variations 246
Snack-Sized Back Attitude 246
   Getting set 247
   The movement 247
   Do's and don'ts 247
   Variations 247
Snack-Sized Ballet Lunges 247
   Getting set 248
   The movement 248
   Do's and don'ts 248
   Variations 248
Snack-Sized Parallel Thighs 248
   Getting set 248
   The movement 249
   Do's and don'ts 249
   Variations 249

Snack-Sized Battements 249
    Getting set 249
    The movement. 250
    Do's and don'ts. 250
    Variations 250
Snack-Sized Side Lifts 250
    Getting set 250
    The movement. 250
    Do's and don'ts. 251
    Variations 251
Snack-Sized Push-Ups at the Counter, Chair, or Couch. 251
    Getting set 251
    The movement. 251
    Do's and don'ts. 252
    Variations 252

PART 4: THE PART OF TENS 253

CHAPTER 15: Ten Important Barre Exercises 255
Pliés 255
Parallel Thigh Work 256
Back Attitude 256
Side Leg Lifts 257
Lunges. 257
Relevés 257
Core C-Curve 258
Planks (Modified or Full) 258
Balance Hold 259
Fold-Over Stretch. 259

CHAPTER 16: Ten Ways to Supercharge Your Workout 261
Breathe on Purpose 261
Warm Up Like You Mean It. 262
Make Small Moves Count. 262
Train Your Focus, Not Just Your Muscles 263
Stop Chasing Perfection. 263
Use Your Core for Everything 263
Respect Recovery. 263
Stack Your Habits with Movement Snacks. 264
Fuel Simply and Eat Mindfully 264
Finish Strong, Then Let It Go 264

CHAPTER 17: **Ten Questions to Ask When Choosing a Class or Instructor**..265

Do I Feel Welcome Here?...266

Does the Instructor Explain Things Clearly?.....................266

Are Modifications Offered and Normalized?.....................266

Is There Room for Fun as Well as Fundamentals?...........267

Is the Pace Something I Can Grow Into?..........................267

Does the Class Feel Encouraging Rather than Competitive?.......267

Are Warm-Ups and Cooldowns Taken Seriously?...........267

Does the Instructor Have Experience and Curiosity?.........268

Can I See Myself Coming Back?..268

How Do I Feel When I Walk Out?......................................268

INDEX..271

Introduction

Welcome to the world of Barre! This book is your friendly, no-nonsense guide to the strength and conditioning workout inspired by classical dance training, Pilates, and functional movement. Designed to build strength, balance, and endurance through small, controlled exercises, Barre is a truly athletic discipline that challenges the body in highly efficient ways while remaining open to everyone. You do not need a dance background, perfect posture, or a special setup at home — and you definitely don't need your own barre. What you do need is curiosity and a willingness to work with your body as it is today. Inside these pages, I show you how Barre works, why it works, what it does for your body, and how to make it work for you. Expect smart training, a little sweat, some shaky muscles, and plenty of encouragement along the way.

In many ways, Barre is all about the plot twist. It looks precise, controlled, and quietly powerful, but it often leaves people scratching their heads and wondering how something so measured can be so effective! At its core, Barre is a low-impact strength and conditioning workout designed to be accessible to everyone. It takes ideas developed in elite movement training and makes them usable, practical, and surprisingly transformative.

By working muscles under sustained tension and emphasizing alignment and posture, Barre improves muscular endurance, balance, and coordination, which is why people often report feeling taller, stronger, and better conditioned even after a short time.

About This Book

This book is here to guide you through a Barre workout in a way that feels supportive, clear, and doable. Whether you are brand new, returning after time away, or simply curious about what all the fuss is about, you are in the right place. Barre is a truly athletic training practice that prioritizes control, alignment, and endurance, and when you understand how it works, it becomes one of the most effective ways to build strength, balance, and confidence in your body. Research consistently shows that this kind of low-impact, high-focus training supports joint health, postural strength, and long-term physical resilience.

I grew up dancing, spent years as a professional dancer, trained as a Pilates instructor, and eventually fell in love with Barre because it brought together everything I believed in: smart movement; small, precise work; and big results that really add up over time. From my guest room, I went on to build Xtend Barre, a global studio brand, pivot to online classes, and create a community of people who show up for themselves regularly, even when life is busy.

This book is an invitation to move your body in a way that feels strong, intelligent, and empowering. You do not need a barre. You do not need a dance background. You do not need to be flexible or coordinated. You do not need a tutu (but you do you!). You just need a willingness to start.

Foolish Assumptions

I've made a few assumptions about you, and I want to get them out in the open right away. You might be brand new to Barre, curious but unsure whether it is really for you. You might have tried a class before and been surprised by how challenging it felt. Or you might already move regularly and be looking for a smarter, more sustainable, low-impact way to build strength.

I assume you are working out at home, not in a studio. You do not need a barre to do these exercises. You may occasionally use something nearby for balance, like a sturdy chair, a kitchen island, or a yoga stick, but even that is optional. This book is designed to meet you where you are, using simple setups that fit real homes and real lives.

You may also have wondered whether Barre can really be effective because of its ballet and dance roots; isn't it all tutus and sparkles? I get it; that is a common assumption. What often gets missed is that dancers are highly trained elite athletes known for their strength, control, and incredible endurance, and Barre borrows thoughtfully from that tradition. The movements are small and precise by design, helping you build deep, lasting strength in a way that is both intelligent and accessible.

Most importantly, I assume that you are a human with a body, not a fitness stereotype. This book is not just for people who already feel fit, flexible, or coordinated. It is for anyone who wants to feel stronger, steadier, and more confident over time. Like almost everything good in this life, Barre rewards consistency, curiosity, and effort, not perfection.

Icons Used in This Book

Throughout this book, icons in the margins highlight certain types of valuable information that call out for your attention. Here are the icons you'll encounter and a brief description of each.

The Tip icon points you to information that helps you perform the exercises correctly or gives you a little extra advice along the way.

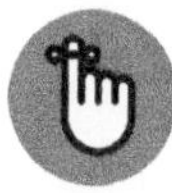

Remember icons mark the information that's especially important to know, especially when you're in the middle of a workout.

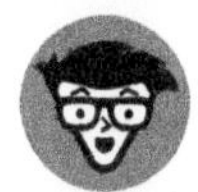

The Technical Stuff icon marks information of a highly technical nature that you can normally skip over, unless, like me, you like knowing the nitty-gritty details!

The Warning icon marks important information to be aware of to prevent injuries and to keep your Barre experience a positive one.

Beyond the Book

In addition to the abundance of information and guidance related to Barre that we provide in this book, you get access to even more help and information online at Dummies.com. Check out this book's online Cheat Sheet. Just go to www.dummies.com and search for "Barre Workouts For Dummies Cheat Sheet."

Where to Go from Here

Although this book is designed for you to move through it in order, building your understanding and confidence along the way, you are always welcome to start wherever you feel most comfortable. Jump in! Every workout includes clear how-to instructions so you can safely follow along, even if, like me, you can't help but jump ahead.

Many readers enjoy taking a little time to learn the central Barre movements and their names first so that they can perform them with confidence during the workouts. Others prefer to begin with a shorter session or a "movement snack" and build from there. However you choose to explore the book, just be sure to warm up first and move at your own pace. Barre meets you where you are and supports you as you go.

1

Getting Started with Barre Workouts

Discover what a Barre workout is, where it comes from, and why it works.

Review how each part of the body plays a role in a Barre workout.

Understand the Barre vocabulary so that you'll know what your instructor is talking about when you hear phrases like "neutral spine," "close your ribs," or "find your C-curve."

Walk through the stages of a Barre workout and discover how to stay motivated and consistent.

Get to know the main moves of a Barre workout and the classical ballet positions they are based on.

Chapter **1**

Stepping Up to the Barre: A Barre Primer

This chapter gives you the lowdown on what Barre actually is — where it comes from, what it looks like in action, and why it works. You discover how small, mindful ballet-inspired movements deliver big results, no prima ballerina background (or wall-mounted barre) required.

What Is a Barre Workout?

Barre is a ballet-inspired workout that's low-impact but seriously high-intensity. It blends the precision of Pilates, the flow of yoga, and the focused discipline of professional dance training into one workout that builds strength, stamina, and flexibility. Don't let the small movements fool you — Barre challenges deep stabilizing muscles you didn't even know you had. It improves your posture, tones your entire body, and sharpens your mind–body connection, all without a single jump or jarring impact. In this book, you will learn the classic moves, follow warm-up and full-workout sequences, and quickly feel confident of the benefits of this iconic (and truly effective) fitness method.

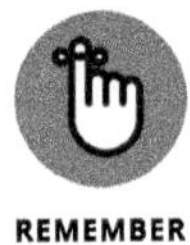

Barre is more than a class or workout; it's movement that strengthens you physically and mentally. It shows you what you are capable of and leaves you feeling empowered, energized, and motivated to take on life with a new level of intention.

Now, the barre itself — the wall-fixed, stationary handrail used for warmups in ballet-training and dance studios around the world — is where the name of this workout derives. But here's the thing: Barre is most definitely not just for dancers. And you most definitely don't need a wall-fixed barre to do it (more on that in a moment).

Barre may be performed in a studio or at home on an exercise mat, barefoot or in grip socks, and occasionally with light hand weights, resistance bands, or a Barre or Pilates ball. Workouts consist of a warm-up, then a series of targeted and challenging exercises that focus on the upper body and arms, the core, abductors, thighs, legs, and feet, and a delicious cooldown at the end to promote flexibility and mobility. With consistency, you'll achieve lean muscle tone, incredible stamina and flexibility, and feel nothing short of amazing.

Ballet-inspired exercise

As Barre borrows from the art of ballet training via Pilates and yoga, you will learn classic ballet moves like pliés, arabesque, and battements (don't worry if this all sounds French to you; we cover how to do all these moves in Chapter 5), and improve your endurance using your own bodyweight via repetitions to challenge the body in targeted ways.

A series of small moves with big results

Many of my clients who are brand-new to Barre workouts are surprised by how quickly they see — and feel — the results. How can such small moves, seemingly simple techniques, and graceful positions deliver toned limbs, a stronger core, improved flexibility, and make their muscles shake like they're bench-pressing 100 pounds? How can such a low-impact workout be so deeply effective at burning fat? And why are these hand weights so light?

"Barre . . . has a reputation for being deceptively hard — all those tiny movements can add up to a rigorous workout," noted *The New York Times* in 2025.

The power of Barre is that, even though the moves can seem small and the weights are light, it's truly a full-body workout. Through a series of targeted and compound movements, a Barre workout focuses on both individual muscles and muscle groups throughout the body. Barre also gives special focus to those smaller muscles that might not otherwise get activated, which tends to promote a more toned, stronger physique. Targeting those muscles — through isometric holds, changing positions, lots of repetitions, sometimes with light weights, a ball, or resistance bands — means those small moves deliver big results.

There is a reason dancers' bodies are so startlingly strong relative to their body mass, and Barre workouts owe much to this much-loved tradition.

Isometric holds

Isometric exercises are static holds in specific positions for a set period. Think wall sits, glute bridges, and planks; in Barre workouts, this is seen in various exercises where we hold the position before or after the movement. These holds activate muscles or muscle groups without moving. Where a biceps curl lengthens (eccentric contraction) and shortens (concentric contraction) your biceps, an isometric exercise is a completely still, static contraction. A Barre workout combines both movement and still moments of isometric exercise to build strength and control.

A QUICK HISTORY OF BARRE

We can thank dance icon Lotte Berk (1913–2003), drawing on a century of classical ballet training and modern expressionist technique, for starting what we now know as Barre. German-born and trained, Lotte's celebrated career found a home in London, England, when she and her husband fled in 1938 on the eve of the Second World War. In 1959, she devised a fitness system for women — a series of dance-based exercises — that soon became the fitness craze of London in the Swinging Sixties. From her basement studio in the city's theater district, Lotte's rumored clientele included celebrities like supermodel Yasmin Le Bon, Joan Collins, and Barbra Streisand. "While Vidal Sassoon did the hair and Mary Quant made the clothes, Lotte Berk took care of the body," wrote *The Times* in 2003.

Like the very best ideas, Lotte's approach was so much to do with perspective. She looked at ballet and dance training in a new way and turned what had been a specialized, elite pursuit into something new and exciting — and open to everyone.

After its success in London, the Lotte Berk Method studio opened in New York City in 1971, and later, other fitness thought-leaders were inspired to create their own barre- and ballet-based classes.

(continued)

(continued)

With my own background as a professional dancer, Pilates instructor, and private fitness coach, and after training hundreds and hundreds of wonderful clients, I think of Barre as the perfect workout. I created the Xtend Method in 2008, opened studios internationally, pivoted to digital classes, and now there's a whole Xtend community of women taking part in online classes, group discussions, and supporting each other. They're the best Barre-friends ever!

Understanding the Fundamentals

Before you jump into your first plié, it helps to understand the core principles that make Barre so effective. From alignment and isometric holds to dealing with the famous "Barre shake," this section breaks down the aims and building blocks of every great Barre workout.

Think of a full Barre workout as incorporating four pillars, or the four S's: Strength, Stamina, Stretch, and Stability.

Strength

You'll be challenging and building strength through resistance, using your body-weight (or occasionally light weights or resistance bands) in moves like Parallel Pliés, Fold-Overs, and C-Curve Abs. (I cover how to do the perfect C-Curve in Chapter 9.) As with all strength-building, your strength will grow when combined with a healthful diet and enough protein (and enough calories in general), good hydration, and skillful sleep.

Stamina

You'll be challenging and improving your stamina, and you'll be able to measure this in your ability to hold positions for longer and with better form, increasing the number of repetitions you're able to do before fatigue, and in the ability and desire to take on longer and more intense workouts. It's a subtle power that grows and is useful in every area of your life.

Stretch

Much like yoga and Pilates, Barre workouts contain a stretch component — it's baked into many of the exercises — that supports general mobility, flexibility, and muscle health, and helps prevent muscle tightness (which, if ignored, can cause injury). Chapter 11 covers active stretching exercises.

Stability

Your ability to maintain a stable center — particularly in your core and pelvis — will start to improve, as a complex network of muscles learn to activate instinctively. Exercises like second cardio, battements, and passé presses, where you move your limbs away from your core, challenge your ability to maintain stability — and it's this challenge that truly improves it. Outside your Barre workouts, your overall balance will improve, which is especially important as we age.

Why You Don't Need a Wall-Mounted Barre

In traditional ballet training, the barre is there for occasional support, and dancers are encouraged to move as if it's not there at all; their fingers brush or tap the barre rather than grip it like their life depends on it!

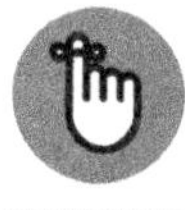

In-studio classes may make clever use of a wall-fixed barre, but many don't, and the exercises in this book do not require one at all.

REMEMBER

If you do need a little extra help with balance, consider an exercise stick (sometimes called a yoga stick or stretching stick). These tools are often made of wood and sometimes have a grip on one end. Or you can simply use the back of your couch, a barstool, or any sturdy surface (around hip height) to support your movement.

TIP

You Don't Have to Be a Dancer — In Fact, Far from It

I trained as a dancer throughout my childhood and teen years and performed professionally into my mid-20s, and let me tell you: We were athletes! Don't be fooled by the tutus and glitter — I trained at least five days a week, took part in endless competitions; it was grueling (and I loved every minute of it). But so much of the art of dance is born from a series of classic moves, performed gracefully with strength and full-out intention. Those moves, performed again and again, improve fitness and flexibility, stamina and strength, and it soon became clear to me that dance-inspired workouts would gift the same strong and confident physique to just about anyone.

Barre is open to all fitness levels and abilities, from people in the process of building or rebuilding their confidence, losing weight, overcoming illness, or entering a new phase of life, from first timers right through to amateur and elite athletes, and, yes, dancers. This is something I truly love about Barre: It really is for everyone! You can take it slow and steady, or — like in my own classes — enjoy a high tempo, dynamic workout knowing both routes mix cardio, strength, endurance, and flexibility.

Practicing Barre for a Lifetime

As Barre draws so generously from ballet, a dance practice that is centuries old, it has incredible longevity. From strengthening the mind-body connection to maintaining mobility and even relieving stress, Barre can truly be in your life for years to come.

Mind-body movement

Mind-body movement might sound a little crystals-and-chakras, but it's a form of exercise that is based in neurology. It pays to familiarize yourself with your body, muscles, and joints, and develop the ability to visualize how they all work together.

Focusing — that is, thinking about — how your body moves and turning on different muscles and muscle groups, truly helps with control. For example, if we mindlessly lift our arms, we aren't truly focusing on *how* we are engaging our muscles to create a certain movement. When mindfully thinking through each movement as we do it, we can often get more bang for our buck out of every rep. Make the most of your efforts by truly focusing your mind on engaging those muscles to your fullest capacity.

Sustainable strength and mobility

Building strength and mobility in a sustainable way comes from consistency, and consistency comes from showing up, harnessing the motivation to roll out your exercise mat, performing your moves, and entering your personal challenge zone (more on that in Chapter 5). As motivation can sometimes be a little elusive, to help, workouts should be easy to set up, fun to do, challenging, and effective. Luckily, Barre is all these things!

Barre's simple setup — just an exercise mat, light weights, resistance bands, exercise ball — challenging moves, and quickly gained results, make staying motivated easy. And while just one Barre workout will leave you feeling strong, sweaty, and at least six feet tall, consistency will create a sustainable improvement in strength and mobility. To read more about the equipment you need, as well as how to stay motivated, check out Chapter 4.

Low impact, high intensity

With its mindful, fluid movements, Barre's naturally low-impact approach is incredibly gentle on joints and tendons, making it the perfect workout for those with arthritis and joint issues. While high-impact exercise has its benefits, low-impact workouts like Barre are generally safer, with a low chance of injury (and they're generally apartment-friendly, too).

But the true power of Barre is that, while it is low-impact, it is also high-intensity and aerobic, steadily activating your cardiovascular system, your muscles, and your whole body. You'll feel challenged and end up with an incredible sense of accomplishment — and who doesn't want that?

Natural stress reliever

All exercise is a stress reliever, helping regulate stress hormones and promote calm and a positive sense of self, but — and I might be biased here — there is something special about Barre. The mental component, learning and maintaining new moves, being hyper-aware of your physicality, growing stronger and more flexible, truly focuses and calms the mind. Barre takes you "out of your head" and into your body. What's more, in 2025, a small study by researchers at Pusan National University in Korea found that senior women who combined regular Barre workouts with walking experienced positive physiological effects: Stress and depression were lowered, and even the immune system got a boost.

Adding Modifications and Progressions

Each exercise in Part 2 of this book details both modifications to help you get the most out of each move and progressions to push yourself a little further. Both are equally smart options. While Barre is open to everyone — no matter your fitness level or physical abilities — not every aspect of every move will be achievable for everyone all the time. (I am a huge fan of modifying during my personal workouts.)

If you're recovering from an injury or have mobility issues (the most common challenges are knees, the lower back, and the neck and shoulders), the smart move is to modify — just make the move a little easier. Paying attention to your body, knowing your own limits, and being honest with yourself when you could push just a little further are integral.

Combining Barre with Other Forms of Exercise

Barre is a truly effective cross-training exercise, perfect for high-impact sports fans, from runners to weight trainers, to help further condition their physiques. Combining exercise types like this and allowing for some contrast in your own fitness activities really pays off. The American Heart Association (AHA) agrees. Drawing on the Physical Activity Guidelines for Americans by the U.S. Department of Health and Human Services, Office of Disease Prevention and Health Promotion, the AHA recommends 150 minutes a week of moderate-intensity aerobic activity, or 75 minutes of vigorous aerobic activity per week, or — better still — a combination of both. Add moderate- to high-intensity muscle-strengthening activity (such as resistance or weights) to at least two days per week, and you're winning! For even more ways to supercharge your Barre workout, see Chapter 16.

Chapter **2**

Reviewing the Barre Body

I n this chapter, you get to know your body from head to toe. You explore how each part plays a role in your Barre practice, which will, in turn, help you target the right muscle groups and avoid injury, from spinal alignment to foot stability and everything in between.

Knowing Your Body from Top to Toe

We receive a continuous stream of information from our sensory receptors and from our skin, joints, and muscles, which helps us move around the world without constantly thinking about it. The incredible processes that guide our movement are called proprioception and kinesthesia — and we barely know they're happening. But developing an awareness of your body and your connection to your physicality not only improves your proprioception and kinesthesia, but it's also essential when learning new ways of moving. You can improve both of these processes by expanding your knowledge of how the body works and through focused physical movement.

Proprioception is your body's ability to sense where it is in space, while *kinesthesia* is your awareness of movement as it happens. Together, they help you balance, coordinate, and move with control, even without looking.

The benefits of really getting to know how your body works are jaw-dropping, from better balance to improved mood, and even a better relationship with chronic pain. Start by getting to know your body from top to toe.

Head, Neck, and Spine

Let's start right at the top, from how you should hold your head, to the impressive mechanical power of the neck, to the S-shaped curve of the spine.

Head

When you are sitting upright or standing, your head weighs around 10 to 12 pounds, but its relative weight on your neck increases when you tilt it (like staring down at a laptop screen or scrolling on your phone, perhaps) or lean it forward or backward. Moving your head like this for prolonged periods puts strain on your neck and spine. Ideally, your head should rest comfortably along the midline of your body, with your ears in line with your shoulders, and with a sense of elevation — stretching softly to the sky. Try to maintain this position in both your Barre workouts and everyday life, from sitting at your desk to driving a car.

Neck

The weight of your head rests on seven cervical vertebrae, which are bony segments that form the smallest and uppermost part of the spine. Our necks are packed full of complex structures — nerves, blood vessels, and muscle groups — and while Barre helps develop neck stability, strength, and mobility, your neck should feel supported and relaxed throughout your workout.

If you start to feel strain in your neck during a workout, try interlacing your fingers and placing them at the base of your skull to very gently offer support, or use a folded towel, yoga block, or pillow to support your neck during supine abdominal work.

Spine

The spine, with its natural S-shape, is made up of an interconnected network of 24 vertebrae and is divided into three main sections: the cervical spine, the thoracic spine, and the lumbar spine.

Cervical spine

At the top is the cervical spine — your neck — which is made up of seven vertebrae, including two special vertebrae that allow for rotation and a curve, like a backward C-shape.

Thoracic spine

The cervical spine is connected to the thoracic spine, which is in the middle part of your back. The thoracic spine is made up of 12 vertebrae that sit in an open C-shape and connect to your ribs. Vertebrae are thinner in the thoracic section, which means the thoracic spine doesn't allow for quite as much movement as both the cervical section and the lumbar section, the lower back.

Lumbar spine

The lumbar section of your spine, with its backward C-shape, is made up of five (or sometimes six) vertebrae that sit above a fusion of many bones at the base that make up the sacrum. The lumbar spine is connected to the pelvis, and in Barre, you'll be using your lumbar spine for pelvic tilts and other movements.

ACHIEVING A NEUTRAL SPINE

A neutral spine is what we call good posture, something all dancers are great at. Standing tall (rather than "standing straight") allows your spine to maintain its natural S-shape while keeping your core gently switched on.

To achieve a neutral spine, position your hips above your knees and your knees in line with your ankles. Tilt your pelvis forward, then backward, and then let it rest in between those two positions. Stack your ribs over your pelvis (we tend to let our pelvis lean back, so be mindful of this) and gently reach the top of your head to the ceiling. Of course, Barre requires you to bend and rotate your whole body, but try to allow for a neutral spine as your default.

Shoulders and Arms

Your shoulders are ball-and-socket joints, meaning their mobility is off the charts! In fact, your shoulders have more potential movement ability than any other joint in the body, and Barre makes full use of this fact with its fluid, mindful, and powerful moves.

Elevation and depression

Shoulder or scapular elevation is the upward movement of the shoulder blades. Shrug, bringing your shoulders up to your ears, and you'll be performing a shoulder elevation.

Scapular depression is the opposite; it's when the shoulder blades drop back down to their resting position. Your traps, or trapezius muscles, are the focus, and it's here where many of us tend to hold tension. Do a few elevations and depressions now, to loosen up your traps.

Protraction and retraction

Protraction and retraction use a different set of muscles: the pectoralis major and serratus anterior. Roll your shoulders forward, separating your shoulder blades for a protraction, and then bring your shoulder blades together, allowing your chest to puff out with an arch in your back for a retraction.

Core

Disciplines like Pilates and yoga are known for their focus on the body's core, and Barre is no different. While a strong, reliable core is key for professional dancers, it's also essential for everyday movements, like picking something off the floor and lacing up your sneakers, to driving a car and unloading the dishwasher. Let's go deep into the core.

The "six pack" (yes, you probably have one!)

We all have a set of abdominal muscles called the *rectus abdominis*, arranged into two connected muscle bands that run vertically down either side of the abdomen. Running across these muscle bands are several bands of connective tissue (fascia) that, once toned, give a visible shape to what we call our "abs." A quirk of the human body is that you are born with a set number of these bands. Most of us have three on each side, creating a "six pack," but others have more or less, creating two, four, or even eight or ten "packs."

Obliques

Your obliques are a large muscle group that runs internally and externally on the side of your rectus abdominis muscles and extends down into your hip joints. They help control twisting and turning movements. Think of them as a corset or stabilizing girdle for your back and pelvis (more on the pelvis later).

Transverse abdominis

The transverse abdominis is a deep abdominal muscle that connects the front of your abdomen to the sides of your body. It helps provide stability and strength to the entire core area (and, if strong, will help define your rectus abdominis).

Pelvis

Considered part of your core, the pelvis connects the top and bottom halves of your body and is laced with powerful muscles alongside organs and joints. The female pelvis is shaped slightly differently from the male pelvis and has some unique structures and ligaments, but everyone can benefit from pelvic stability, from strength and flexibility in your hips to your pelvic floor (the supportive "sling" of muscle that connects the sacrum to the pubic bone at the front).

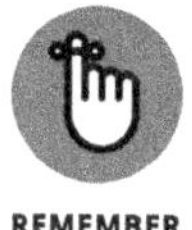

Barre helps develop pelvic stability through tilts and lower-body exercises that target a wide range of musculature.

REMEMBER

Butt

Barre is brilliant for your butt, and no wonder, as your rear just happens to house the largest muscle group in the human body. With a strong focus on the lower body, Barre exercises like Back Attitude and side lifts help develop your gluteus maximus, gluteus medius, and gluteus minimus — your glutes — three separate muscles known for their power and strength. Your genes determine much of the shape of your butt, but anyone can work to strengthen and tone this area.

Knees, Ankles, and Feet

The lower body contains a series of hardworking joints and muscle groups, all of which love to move — but only in the correct way.

Knees

The knee is a complex joint. It is the largest hinge joint in the body, connecting the shinbone to the thighbone. It is housed in protective ligaments, cushioned with cartilage, shock absorbers, and capped with the patella bone.

During workouts, it is important to override any tendency to lock your knees in place. Instead, keep them very slightly "soft" by activating your muscles rather than just relying on the joints themselves. Future you will thank you! Maintaining good alignment from your ankle to your knee and from your knee to your hip is also essential (you explore perfect knee placement in Chapter 3). When doing moves like pliés, let your knees follow the direction of your foot. As a low-impact exercise, Barre is a go-to for many of my clients with knee issues.

There's your home set-up to consider, too: A thin yoga mat on a hard floor may not give you the support you need, so consider using a thicker exercise mat, laying an extra mat on top of another, or folding your mat when doing certain moves.

Be careful not to hyperextend your knees. *Hyperextending* is when a joint bends beyond its usual limit, stretching ligaments and causing pain.

Ankles and feet

In terms of bones (28!), joints (33!), ligaments, muscles, and nerve endings, the feet are one of the most complex parts of the anatomy, built for shock absorption, balance, and support.

The ankles consist of three bones, reinforced by ligaments, that can move in two main directions and are built to withstand an incredible amount of pressure. In Barre, you'll be stretching and strengthening these incredibly complex body parts.

Developing natural foot alignment helps maintain happy feet. Here's what you need to know:

>> **The four points:** Think of the foot as being divided into four points: two at the front, behind the big toe and the little toe, and two in the heel, on the inside

and the outside. Try for a neutral distribution of weight between all four points.

- **Pronation:** This is when you tend to carry more weight on the inside of the foot, behind the big toe, and inside the heel. Pronation can cause problems in the foot, ankle, and right up the legs to the knees, hips, and pelvis — even your back. Barre can help you maintain a more equal balance.

- **Supination:** The opposite of pronation, supination is when your weight tends to concentrate on the outside of the foot behind the little toe and the outside of the heel. It can cause the same problems as pronation. Barre can help you maintain a more equal balance.

- **Ankle and foot stability:** All your weight is carried in your feet and ankles, so it follows that they need to be as strong and as supple as possible. There is a focus on this area of the body in Barre, and you'll feel its benefits in no time at all.

Muscle System

Put simply, your muscles help you move! Skeletal muscles are dynamic and attach to your bones via tendons, and there are more than 650 of them in the human body. When you move with intention — that is, really thinking about what you're doing — you are asking those muscles to work together with purpose rather than on autopilot. This kind of focused movement improves coordination, strength, and efficiency, which is why Barre emphasizes control, precision, and awareness rather than rushing through exercises while you're thinking about what you need to pick up from the store later. Dancers train this way because intentional movement creates better outcomes with less wasted effort, and the same approach benefits everyone in almost any fitness discipline.

Your muscle system also works closely with fascia, the web of connective tissue that surrounds and supports your muscles, organs, and joints. Fascia helps transmit force and allows muscles to glide smoothly against one another, which is essential for fluid, pain-free movement. It is naturally lubricated with hyaluronan, the same substance often found in skincare products, and it responds best to regular, varied movement, which is why warm-ups are so important. When you move mindfully and consistently, as you do in Barre, you support both your muscles and your fascia, helping your body stay resilient, mobile, and well connected.

Chapter **3**

Learning the Terms: Barre Talk

arre has its own vocabulary, and this chapter helps you speak the language. In this chapter, you get familiar with the essential alignment cues, anatomical references, and terms that instructors use to guide movement safely, effectively, and with precision. By the end, you'll know exactly what your instructor (and this book!) is talking about when you hear or read phrases like "neutral spine," "close your ribs," or "find your C-curve." When you understand the language of Barre, you can move with greater focus, safety, and intention. That's what makes these small movements so powerful, and why Barre, once you know how it works, is anything but easy.

The Core: Your Power Center

Everything in Barre begins with your core. The core is more than your abdominal muscles. It includes the deep muscles of your abdomen, the muscles that support your spine, your pelvic floor, and even the muscles around your hips. Together, they create a stable base that allows your limbs to move with control and efficiency. A strong, connected center supports balance, alignment, and every lift or pulse you perform.

This is why the core is often called your *power center*. When it is engaged, movement feels lighter, more coordinated, and more supported. In Barre, you learn to initiate movement from this central system rather than relying on momentum, gravity, or isolated muscle effort. The result is strength that transfers into better posture, improved balance, and greater ease in everyday movement.

To engage your core, brace your abdominals, drawing your belly button in toward your spine. A simple way to reset your core is to inhale, expanding the area below your ribs, lower back, waist, and pelvic floor, then relax everything and exhale, gently holding your stomach muscles in. Keep this subtle (no need to strain!) but strong connection throughout your workout. A good visual is to think of drawing your belly button in toward your spine and up.

Pelvic control

Think of your pelvis as your body's steering wheel. Pelvic control refers to connecting your hips, lower back, and abdominal muscles so that they work together for stable, precise movement. When your pelvis is under control, the rest of your form falls into place.

Over-tucking the pelvis flattens your natural spinal curve, so aim for steady, not stiff.

Posterior tilt

This "tuck" position happens when you draw your tailbone slightly under your pubic bone and toward your belly button, as shown in Figure 3-1. You'll feel your abdominals engage and your lower back lengthen. It's a key move in many Barre positions that builds core awareness and lower-body strength.

Anterior tilt

The opposite of a tuck. Your tailbone tips slightly back, and your seat lifts, as shown in Figure 3-2. It can feel like a small arch in the lower back. Keep this movement controlled and gentle to avoid straining the lumbar area.

If you feel pinching in your back, bring your pelvis closer to neutral.

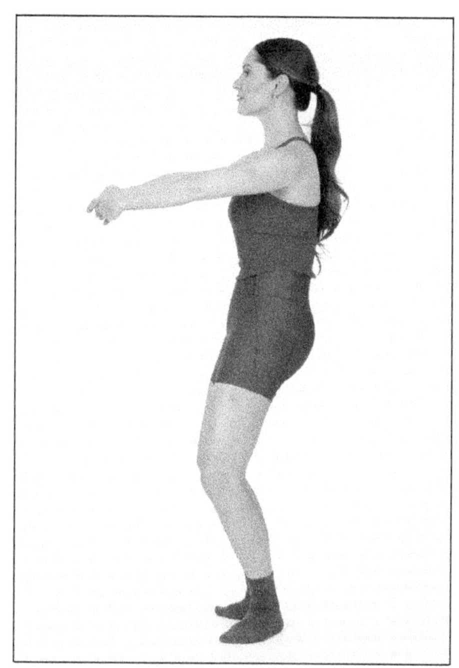

FIGURE 3-1:
Tuck your
tailbone slightly
under your pubic
bone and toward
your belly button.

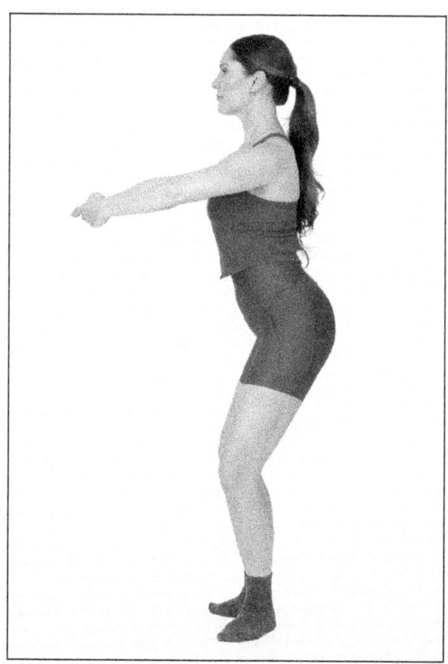

FIGURE 3-2:
The opposite of a
tuck. Your
tailbone tips
slightly back and
your seat lifts.

Neutral pelvis

Think of this as your default position. When your hip bones and pubic bone line up evenly and parallel to the floor, your pelvis is nice and neutral (Figure 3-3). From this balanced position, your body can move efficiently and safely.

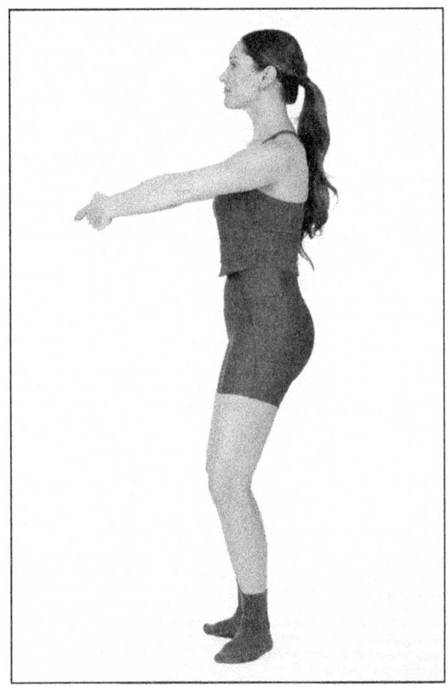

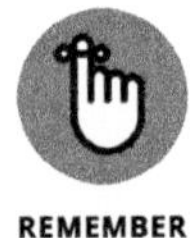

REMEMBER

Most Barre exercises begin with a neutral pelvis. Master this, and your alignment everywhere else improves.

Navel to spine

A classic Barre cue. When I'm teaching, I find myself saying navel to spine countless times a day! It's so easy and easily forgotten. Imagine gently zipping up your abdominals, drawing your belly button toward your spine. This activates your deepest core muscles and gives you that strong, centered feeling from the inside out.

Creating a C-curve

The C-curve is a hallmark of Barre, Pilates, and yoga positions. To create a C-curve, round your spine slightly into a soft "C" shape by tucking your pelvis, engaging your abdominals, and rounding through your upper back. This movement strengthens your core, stretches your spine, and builds incredible endurance.

When creating a C-curve, be mindful not to just collapse your chest. Keep space between your ribs and thighs so you can breathe and stay lifted.

Alignment and Posture: Building the Framework

Barre's high-intensity effects are directly connected to how well you line everything up. And by everything, I mean your head, shoulders, rib cage, spine, pelvis, hips, knees, and feet, all working together as one connected system. When your body is aligned, your muscles can do the job they are meant to do, without unnecessary strain or compensation.

Proper alignment also protects your joints, supports healthy movement patterns, and it really helps prevent injury over time. It also lets you work smarter, not harder. When things are stacked correctly, small movements become far more effective, which is one of Barre's greatest strengths. You may not be moving much, but your body knows exactly what it is doing. Think of alignment as the framework that makes everything else possible. Get that right, and the work feels stronger, safer, and empowering.

Neutral spine

Keeping a neutral spine means maintaining the natural S-curve of your spine, so no flattening or arching. Think of a string gently pulling the crown of your head toward the ceiling as your tailbone reaches down. With a neutral spine, your back feels long, strong, and balanced.

Neutral shoulders and arms

When you hear "neutral shoulders" or "neutral arms," it means you should relax your shoulders, letting them drop slightly back to create a broad, open chest and a long neck. Let your arms stay light but active, extended from the shoulder with control.

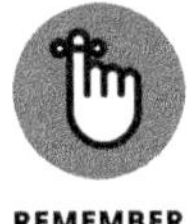

Hunching or shrugging creates tension. Try to keep your shoulders low and your upper body "proud."

Closed ribs

To close your ribs, draw your lower ribs inward toward your center to connect your core and upper body. This stabilizes your spine, improves posture, and helps prevent your ribs from flaring out during movement.

Imagine your ribs as an umbrella: open as you breathe in, close gently as you exhale.

Square off (or box)

You might hear an instructor say something like "square your hips," "keep your shoulders square," or "box it up." This simply means lining up your hips and shoulders so that they face the same direction, like the four corners of a neat little box.

In class, this cue usually shows up during single-leg work or anything that might tempt your body to twist, cheat, or wander off course. Squaring off keeps things as they should be — a reset, if you will. When your hips and shoulders stay aligned, the right muscles do the work, and your joints stay happier. Even though this book doesn't rely heavily on the term, it's a common piece of instructor shorthand. Think of it as a friendly reminder to stay centered, balanced, and not let one side of your body take over.

The midline

The midline refers to an imaginary line that runs centrally through your body from the top of your head to the floor. Drawing energy toward this line improves stability and balance, especially during single-leg or one-arm work. Many exercises have you move your limbs mindfully across it.

The Lower Body: Strength, Balance, and Power

Your lower body is where Barre really earns its rep. Those tiny, controlled movements build strength, balance, and power while reinforcing alignment from the ground up. This is also where many people first notice what is often called the *Barre burn*.

The Barre burn is the warm, intense sensation you feel in a muscle when it has been working continuously under tension. It usually shows up during sustained holds, small pulses, or many sets of slow, controlled movements. This feeling is closely related to the Barre shakes I mentioned in Chapter 1. Both are signs that your muscles are being challenged in a deep, targeted way, particularly in their endurance fibers. In simple terms, the muscle is working hard in a small range, and your nervous system is fully engaged. This sensation should not be confused with any delayed muscle soreness that might occur after pushing yourself too hard.

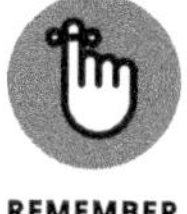

REMEMBER

The burn and the shakes are not something to fear or push through aggressively. They are useful feedback. They tell you that the muscle is doing its job. You can always lessen the intensity by reducing the range of motion, straightening your legs slightly, or taking a brief reset. Barre is about controlled challenge, and never about suffering.

Foot stability and alignment

Your feet are your base of support. Press down through all four corners of each of your feet — just behind the big toe, little toe, and both sides of your heel — while lifting gently through your arches. This improves balance and keeps your knees and hips aligned.

WARNING

Don't curl your toes under. Keep them long and relaxed to strengthen your arches naturally.

Knee placement

Keep your knees tracking directly over your toes. It sounds simple, but this alignment is the difference between strong and sore. Proper placement protects your joints and keeps every plié and squat smooth. Take extra care here, and not just during your Barre workout. Correct placement of the knee will help you in every physical task you do! See Figures 3-4 and 3-5 for examples of correct and incorrect knee placement.

TIP

If you can't see your toes in a plié, shift your weight slightly back. Your glutes will engage more — and your knees will thank you.

FIGURE 3-4: With incorrect knee placement, knees bow inward (a); whereas with correct knee placement, your knees, hip, and toes are in line (b).

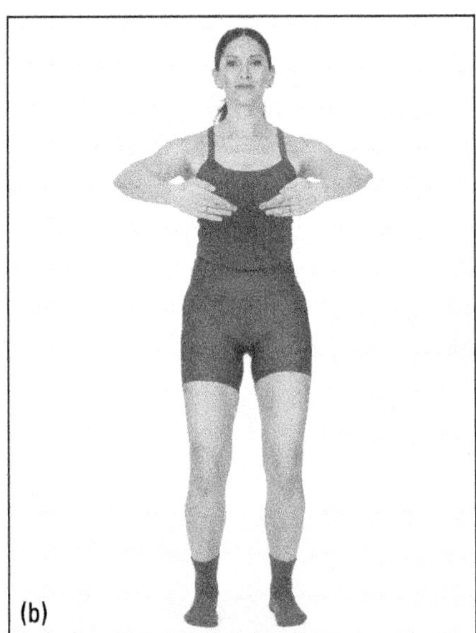

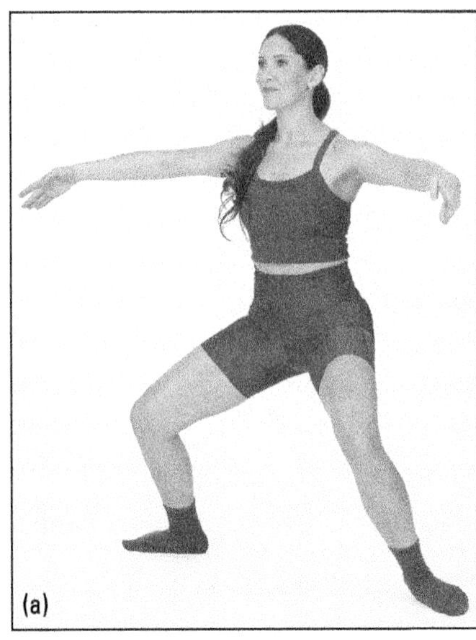

FIGURE 3-5: Bowed knees put strain on the joints (a); whereas with correct knee placement, knees are more vertical (b).

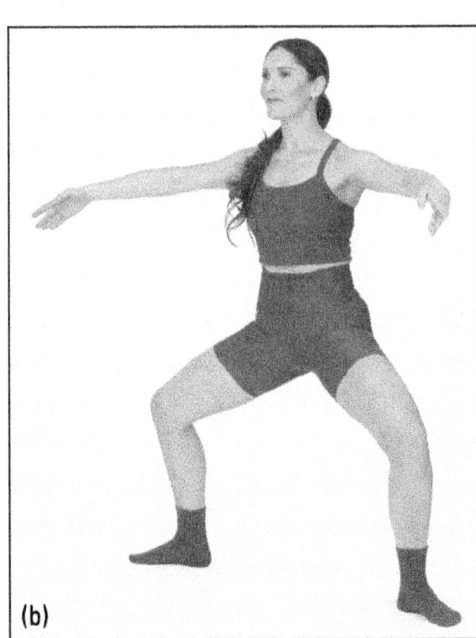

Isometric exercise

Isometric exercise is a type of exercise in which you hold a position while staying active. These holds, sometimes with tiny pulses, fire up muscles without movement, which is why your legs might shake during class. That shake means your muscles are working hard in their smallest range. Barre workouts emphasize isometric exercise to build endurance and strength.

Static stretch

A static stretch refers to a calm, steady stretch that is held for several seconds to improve flexibility and recovery. Breathing deeply during static stretches helps lengthen tight muscles and signals your body to relax.

Movement Mechanics: How You Move

Barre exercises may look like small movements, but the mechanics behind them are deeply effective. Understanding how and why you move ensures each repetition works in your favor. Every motion should come from muscle control, not momentum. When you move with precision, activating specific muscle groups, you'll tone faster and prevent injury.

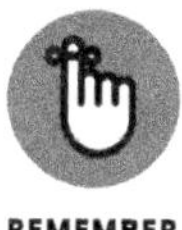

Smaller, slower, and more controlled means better results.

Lift with purpose

Stability doesn't just mean stillness; it means your muscles are working together to keep you steady and feeling strong. Every lift should feel light yet controlled, as if your body is supported from within.

Planes of movement

Your body moves in three main directions. Understanding them helps you move with awareness and balance.

>> **Frontal plane:** Side-to-side motions, like leg lifts or lateral arm reaches.

>> **Sagittal plane:** Forward-and-back movements, such as lunges or hip hinges.

>> **Transverse plane:** Twisting or rotating movements that strengthen your obliques and improve coordination.

Mixing all three planes creates a well-rounded, balanced workout.

Range of motion

Your *range of motion* is how far you can move a joint comfortably and safely. In Barre, smaller often means smarter: Tiny, controlled ranges target the muscles more deeply than big, sweeping movements. Your range of motion is personal to you, so feel free to modify if something doesn't feel quite right.

Avoid hyperextending (locking) your joints. Keep a soft bend in your elbows and knees for protection.

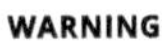

Even when it's your legs that are burning, your upper body and stabilizing muscles are working, too. Barre strengthens the body as a connected system, so don't forget to give your upper body some attention.

Supportive leg or arm

Your supportive leg or arm — the *stabilizer* — is the limb that keeps you balanced and aligned while the other side moves. Though it looks passive, this supportive limb is constantly engaged to hold you steady, firing up sets of muscles reactively to maintain your form as the rest of your body moves.

Working leg or arm

The working leg or arm is the opposite of the stabilizer; it's the limb that is performing the main action: the lift, pulse, or extension. The working limb takes the spotlight, but it really relies on the supportive side for control and precision.

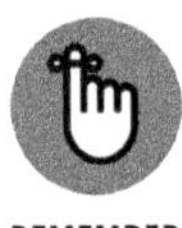

Both sides of your body are always working: the one moving, and the one holding you up. That's why Barre feels like a full-body workout!

Chapter **4**

Preparing for Your First Workout

This chapter shows you how to get set up for success, starting with your very first Barre workout. You discover how to prep your space and what equipment is essential. You then explore what each segment of the workout is designed to do and how to show up for your body in every phase, even when your barre is a kitchen counter or a sturdy chair. You also find out ways to stay motivated and consistent so you can enjoy Barre for a lifetime.

Setting Up Your Space

Before you start plié-ing and pulsing, take a few minutes to prep your environment, gather your equipment, and change into your workout clothes. At-home Barre is about creating space, both physically and mentally, so you can move safely and confidently.

Choose a spot with good lighting and room to move freely. Clear a six-by-six-foot area, if possible, with no obstacles. A thicker exercise mat provides cushioning and a defined workspace. A mirror is incredibly helpful. It helps you check posture and alignment in real time. No need for a studio setup; a full-length mirror propped securely against the wall works beautifully — just make sure it doesn't invade your space to avoid accidents.

Avoid working near rugs that slide, furniture with sharp corners, or slippery floors. If your surface feels slick, lay down your mat or use a towel for traction. I can't stress enough how important it is to properly audit your space and prepare for safety.

Keep your pets and kids clear of your workout space. Barre may be calm, but a wagging tail underfoot is still a trip hazard!

Choosing the right equipment

One of the best things about doing Barre at home is how little equipment you actually need to get started. Barre is built around bodyweight resistance, alignment, and control, not gadgets. That means you can do a very effective workout at home without investing in a full, slick studio setup.

Here is the basic equipment I recommend:

>> A good-quality exercise mat

>> A sturdy chair nearby or a countertop for balance

>> A pair of light hand weights (1 to 3 pounds)

>> A soft, squishy soccer-ball-sized ball or a firm cushion for thigh work

>> A resistance band, if you'd like to level up

>> An exercise stick or yoga stick, if you want a little help with balance

The only truly essential piece of equipment is a good-quality exercise mat. Look for a mat that provides enough cushioning to support your knees, hips, and spine during floor work, but is still firm enough to provide stability during standing exercises, and has online reviews that talk up its grip power. A medium-thickness mat usually works well, offering comfort without feeling unstable. Everything else is optional and meant to enhance the work, not define it.

If you do not have traditional fitness equipment, everyday household items work just as well: filled plastic water bottles instead of weights, a pillow instead of a ball. The goal of Barre is mindful, controlled movement, not collecting a slew of props.

Wearing the right clothes

What you wear during a Barre workout plays a bigger role than you might expect. Fitted clothing, such as leggings and a snug tank or tee, allows you to move freely while also making it easier to see your alignment in the mirror. Because Barre focuses on small, precise movements, being able to see what your hips, knees, and spine are doing helps you make subtle adjustments to improve your form and protect your joints. Fitted clothing is also more comfortable during sustained holds and floor work because nothing bunches up, slides, or twists as you move.

Overall, you need to be comfortable, so it is best to avoid clothing that restricts movement or hides your body position. Jeans, stiff fabrics, or anything with buttons or zippers are a definite no. Baggy tops, oversized sweatshirts, or wide-leg pants can get in the way, ride up, or make it harder to tell if you are aligned correctly. The goal is not to look a certain way, but to feel supported and able to focus fully on the work.

As for hair, it is entirely up to you. If you have long hair, tying it back in a ponytail or bun can make floor work and balance exercises more comfortable, especially when you are lying on your back or moving through planks. That said, there is no strict rule. Choose whatever helps you feel comfortable, focused, and ready to move without distraction.

Upgrading your experience with music

Music sets the mood for your movement. Whether you're into upbeat pop or mellow instrumental, choose tracks that match your pace and keep you energized. My classes focus on tempo, using an uplifting playlist. I suggest trying a set list that gradually builds intensity and then softens toward the end. It helps you flow naturally through your workout.

GRIP SOCKS: YOUR SECRET WEAPON

Grip socks are a must for at-home Barre. They give your feet traction, help prevent slips, and provide gentle arch support. They also keep your toes warm and your movements grounded.

If you prefer to be barefoot, that's fine — just make sure your exercise mat allows for a strong grip, and the floor around you is clean, dry, and not slick.

Consider playing music through a speaker rather than headphones or earbuds so that you can move freely without cords getting in the way or losing a bud mid-move.

Examining the Main Components of a Barre Workout

A Barre workout is low-impact, joint-friendly, and endlessly adaptable. It's gentle on your joints but challenging for your muscles, and it really grows with you. Expect small, precise movements that target strength, balance, and flexibility, all within the space of an exercise mat.

This section walks you through a full at-home Barre workout from your first pulse to your final stretch. You'll often alternate between standing and floor sequences, occasionally using a chair, wall, or nothing at all. There is no jumping, no loud impact, just quiet, focused effort that sneaks up on you (in the very best way). It sets you up nicely for Part 2 of this book, where you learn specific workouts for each of the main components here.

In a Barre workout, small movements don't mean easier — it means you're working with focus and control.

Warming up

Every great workout starts with a proper warm-up. This is your body's gentle wake-up call, getting blood flowing to your muscles, lubricating your joints and fascia, and shifting your focus from the day to your movement. Expect easy shoulder rolls, arm circles, pliés, and leg swings. Keep it light, rhythmic, and mindful. When I warm up, I'm telling my body it's time to move, be challenged, and set my intentions for the workout ahead.

Check your space before you start. Clear away coffee tables, plants, and pets. Your workout area should be free of clutter and large enough for you to extend your arms and legs comfortably in all directions.

Starting with the upper body

Many Barre routines begin by focusing on the upper body using light weights or even just your own resistance. You'll tone your arms, shoulders, and back with small, high-rep movements like pulses, lifts, and squeezes. Even without equipment, you can sculpt strength through control and awareness. Move slowly, engage your muscles, and focus on strong posture. Your posture is your best prop.

Moving to barre (chair) work

No barre? No problem. If you need it, a sturdy chair, countertop, or wall can provide all the support you need during this next segment of a Barre workout. (Remember, in professional ballet training, the barre is there for occasional support — it's not gripped.)

If you are using a chair for support, make sure it is heavy enough or positioned against a wall so that it doesn't tip.

This part of a Barre workout targets your legs and glutes with small, precise movements like pliés, leg lifts, and pulses that challenge balance and stability. You might feel your legs start to shake. It means your stabilizers are firing and you're building long, lean strength — but don't worry, you'll be changing position and focusing on a new muscle group in moments.

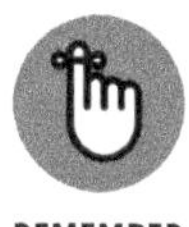

You don't need a barre to do the exercises in this segment, but if you feel more confident with something safe and sturdy nearby, be my guest!

Strengthening your core

The next part of a Barre workout focuses on what Joseph Pilates, the inventor of Pilates, calls the "powerhouse" — the core. Whether you're seated, standing, or down on the mat, your core is the anchor of every move in a Barre workout. You'll practice control rather than crunches, focusing on small, precise contractions that build deep strength and stability. Engage your abdominals by gently drawing your belly button toward your spine, exhale through effort, and try to keep a gentle engagement throughout your workout.

Focusing on floor work

Floor work brings everything together. This is the segment of a Barre workout where you isolate and fine-tune muscles with exercises like glute bridges, side-lying leg lifts, and tabletop core work.

Because you're already warmed up, your body can move more deeply and with more control. Use a mat or towel for comfort, keep your neck in a neutral position, and listen to your body's cues.

A well-performed Barre workout looks fluid and precise, but it's all about focus. By perfecting your form and focusing your attention on the muscle you're working, you activate more fibers and become stronger and faster. Imagine the muscle contracting, visualize its power, and stay present. That's what turns small movements into major results and helps develop calmness and a positive sense of well-being.

Cooling down and stretching

Stretching shouldn't be an afterthought; it's an important and enjoyable finish. The cooldown phase helps your heart rate lower gradually and allows your body to release tension after all that effort.

During the cooldown segment of a Barre workout, slow down, breathe deeply and steadily, and feel your body unwind. It's your time to acknowledge your work and leave your mat feeling calmer (and maybe a little taller) than when you started.

Keep a mirror nearby during stretches, too. It's a great way to spot any lingering tension in your shoulders or posture.

Being Consistent

The secret to progress isn't perfection — it's showing up consistently, even when you don't feel like it. Small, steady effort beats occasional bursts of enthusiasm. Commit to short, regular exercise sessions; even a few 20-minute workouts a week can create real change.

Try these ways to keep your consistency strong:

>> **Schedule your workout like a meeting.** Pick your workout times in advance and protect them.

>> **Keep it short.** Twenty focused minutes beat none.

>> **Track your wins.** A simple check mark on a calendar builds momentum.

>> **Celebrate effort, not outcome.** Showing up is the victory here.

Staying Motivated

Motivation ebbs and flows. That's normal. But the more you do, the more you'll want to do. It's truly a cycle so instead of waiting for inspiration, build habits that carry you through dips in energy.

When motivation is low, try following this cycle, which uses the proven cue–routine–reward structure of habit formation:

>> Prepare your space the night before. Set out your mat, props, or grip socks.

>> Cue your playlist before you start so you're ready to move.

>> Start small. Tell yourself you just need enough get-up-and-go for five minutes — momentum will carry you from there.

>> Revisit your "why." Remind yourself how good it feels when you're done.

The first minute of any exercise routine is always the hardest, but once you're in it, it feels so good! Once you're done, reward yourself (hopefully with something healthful, but you do you!).

Keep a sticky note on your mirror with a short reminder or words of encouragement — something like "strong posture, strong mind." It's amazing how much that small cue can boost motivation.

Marking movements

Marking is a term from the dance world. Dancers mark choreography when they are saving energy or running through the steps in their heads rather than going full out. Translation: The body is moving, but the muscles are not fully committing.

5, 6, 7, 8, GO!

This dancer's countdown is your mental switch. "5, 6, 7, 8" means it's time to focus, connect, and move with intent. Even at home, this countdown brings rhythm and precision to your practice. Cue yourself out loud if you want (I know I do!); it's surprisingly motivating and instantly boosts your energy.

In Barre, marking shows up when you are distracted, tired, or just not feeling it. You go through the shapes, but the intention is missing. And that's okay. Some days are full-out days, and some days are mark-it-and-move-on days. Although Barre works best when you really bring focus and engagement, even a marked workout still counts. If you notice it happening, smile, shrug, take a breath, and rejoin the work at whatever level feels right.

Giving a full-out effort

Full-out effort, on the other hand, is all about intention. If you are giving a full-out effort, you feel every pulse, every squeeze, every breath. When you commit fully — mindfully engaging, even to tiny motions — you get deeper activation, stronger results, and a bigger endorphin payoff.

Full-out is a term from my dancing days. After learning a new routine, breaking it down into a series of small moves, my teacher would ask us to perform the whole thing full out, with everything we had, to the very highest standard we could muster.

In this book, full-out means giving your best energy for today, not perfection. Some days full-out might mean power and sweat; other days it's slow and steady. Either way, consistency compounds. You don't need to go full-out each and every workout session in order to be successful.

Balancing mastery with novelty

Repeating familiar sequences helps you refine your technique and build your confidence. But new challenges, such as adding resistance bands, balance work, or progressions to every exercise in this book, keep your body and brain adapting.

Here's how to balance mastery of your movements with novelty of the exercise:

>> **Get great at the familiar.** Focus on form and precision in moves you already know.

>> **Introduce one new challenge each week.** It can be a new prop, tempo change, or playlist.

>> **Change your setting.** Move to your favorite song, take your workout outdoors, or try a new online class (I'd love to see you in mine!).

>> **Notice progress.** Every tweak helps your body learn something new.

Mixing it up helps keep the spark — and your motivation — alive.

Chapter 5

Getting into Position: The Main Moves

This chapter breaks down the classic positions every Barre workout is made of. You'll learn how to set up the position, how to perform it, and the benefits each position brings to your workout, including, where relevant, a quick nod to the dance world it came from. Get to know these moves, and you'll know exactly what to expect, how the position fits into the world of Barre, and how each section supports your strength and mobility. Get ready to learn classical ballet positions, technical foundations, classical dance movements, dynamic movements, and concepts like the challenge zone.

Classical Ballet Positions

Classical ballet positions are often the starting point for Barre moves. In this section, I define each position and describe what it is, why it matters, and how to do it — just like dancers do!

First position: Feet

This classical ballet stance sets you up with a turned-out foundation that supports strength, stability, and clean alignment for countless barre movements.

What it is

First position is a traditional ballet stance in which your heels touch and your toes turn outward into a natural V-shape, as shown in Figure 5-1.

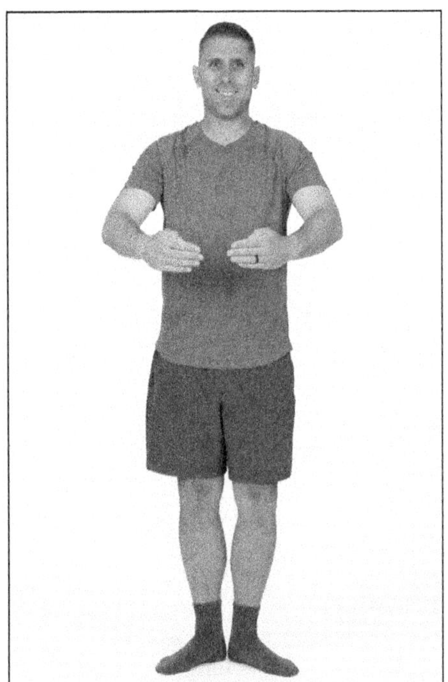

Why it matters

It builds your turnout, posture, and alignment for many barre movements.

How to do it

Placing your feet in first position involves four steps:

1. Stand tall with a neutral spine.

2. Bring your heels together and turn your toes out from your hips.

3. Engage your inner thighs so that your knees line up with your toes.

4. Lift through your center.

Do's and don'ts

» Do keep your turnout coming from your hips.

» Do keep your weight even and maintain a neutral pelvis.

» Don't force your turnout or roll inward on your arches.

Variations

» Try narrow first — only slightly turning out your feet rather than rotating them wide if you want a gentler turnout and more stability. Instead of forcing turnout, you allow your legs to rotate naturally from the hips. For many people new to Barre, narrow first feels more stable and safer than a wide turnout.

» Performing a relevé in first position adds a balance challenge while strengthening your calves and ankles.

A *relevé* is a classic Barre and ballet movement that simply means lifting your heels off the floor, balancing on the balls of your feet. You will find a more detailed breakdown of relevé, including how to do it safely and confidently, later in this chapter.

First position: Arms

This classical ballet arm position helps you create a lifted, graceful shape that supports your posture, balance, and expressive upper-body movement.

What it is

First position is a classical ballet arm position in which your arms form a soft oval in front of your body at rib height (see Figure 5-1).

Why it matters

It promotes your upper-body alignment, core engagement, and graceful transitions.

How to do it

Placing your arms in first position involves three steps:

1. Round your arms softly in front of you.

2. Keep your elbows lifted and your hands facing each other.

3. Relax your shoulders and lift through your sternum.

Do's and don'ts

» Do keep your arms supported from your back.

» Don't let your elbows droop or your shoulders creep up.

Variations

Try lowering or raising your arms slightly if you want to explore different levels of support and expression.

Second position: Feet

This wide, turned-out stance creates a strong base that supports powerful lower-body work and clean classical lines.

What it is

Second position is a classical ballet stance where your feet are wider than your hips, and your toes are turned outward, as shown in Figure 5-2.

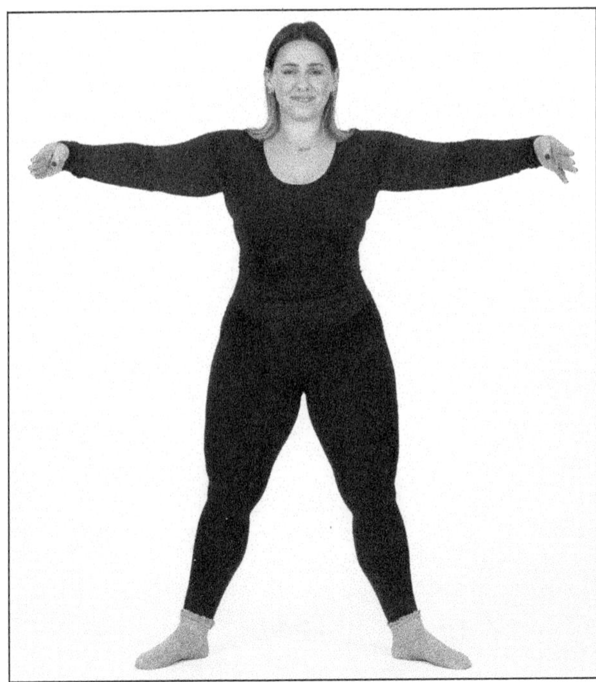

FIGURE 5-2: A classical ballet stance where your feet are wider than your hips and your toes are turned outward.

Why it matters

It gives you stability for pliés, weight shifts, and lateral work.

How to do it

Placing your feet in second position involves three steps:

1. Start with your feet in first position.
2. Step one foot to the side until your feet are wider than hip width.
3. Maintain turnout from your hips.

Do's and don'ts

>> Do keep your weight evenly distributed.

>> Don't over-rotate your feet.

Variations

>> Take a slightly wider stance for deeper leg work.

>> Try a narrower stance if you want more stability.

Second position: Arms

This open, rounded arm position helps you create width, stability, and elegance through your upper body while supporting your balance.

What it is

Second position is a classical ballet arm position in which your arms extend wide and are slightly rounded (see Figure 5-2).

Why it matters

It strengthens your shoulders, opens your chest, and supports your balance.

How to do it

Placing your arms in second position involves three steps:

1. Reach your arms out to your sides at shoulder height.

2. Keep a gentle curve in your elbows and wrists.

3. Relax your shoulders downward.

Do's and don'ts

>> Do keep a gentle lift under your arms.

>> Don't lock your elbows.

Variations

>> Lower the arms if you want less shoulder engagement.

>> Lift your arms slightly higher to increase upper-body work.

Low fifth and high fifth positions: Arms

These two classical arm shapes help you build strength and control through a full range of motion in your shoulders and upper back.

What it is

Low fifth position and high fifth position are two classical ballet positions in which your arms are rounded low (low fifth) or overhead (high fifth).

Why it matters

They improve your upper-body coordination and help you move smoothly between arm pathways.

How to do it

Placing your arms in either low or high fifth position involves two steps:

1. Keep your arms softly rounded.

2. For low fifth position, hold your hands near hip height (Figure 5-3), and for high fifth position, hold your arms overhead without lifting your shoulders (Figure 5-4).

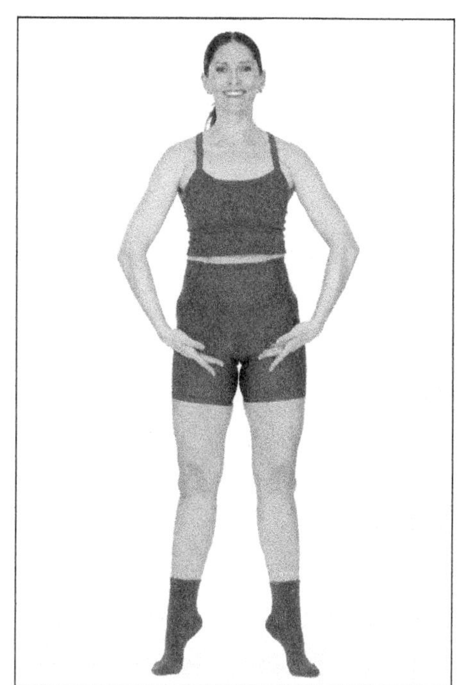

FIGURE 5-3:
Low fifth position:
With your arms
softly rounded,
hold your hands
near hip height
(shown here with
optional
heel lifts).

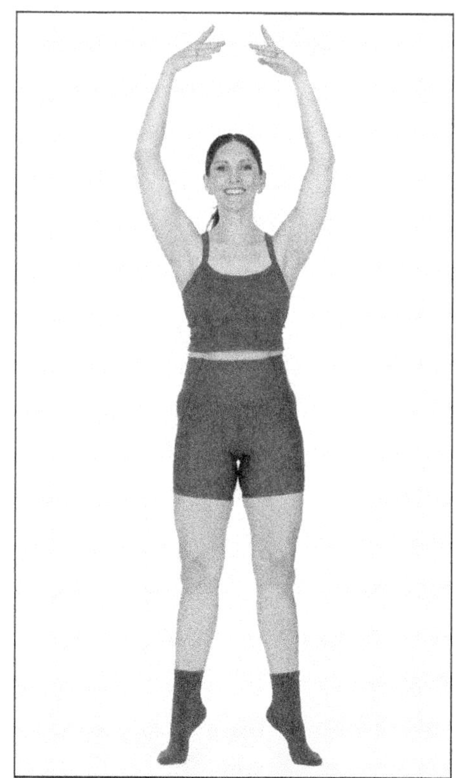

FIGURE 5-4:
High fifth
position: Hold
your arms
overhead,
keeping your
shoulders relaxed
(shown here with
optional
heel lifts).

Do's and don'ts

>> Do support the shape from your back.

>> Don't collapse your wrists.

Variations

>> Move between low fifth, first, second, and high fifth positions to build smooth transitions.

>> Try holding high fifth a little longer to build endurance in your shoulders.

Port de bras

This flowing ballet movement helps you develop graceful arm pathways while coordinating your posture, breath, and upper-body control.

What it is

Port de bras is a classical ballet term meaning "carriage of the arms," referring to smooth transitions between positions.

Why it matters

It improves your flow, expression, posture, and upper-body mobility.

How to do it

This movement involves three steps:

1. Move your arms fluidly from one position to the next.

2. Initiate movement from your back muscles.

3. Coordinate with your breath.

Do's and don'ts

>> Do let your arms travel smoothly.

>> Don't rush or let your shoulders lift.

Variations

>> Try a port de bras movement through first, second, and fifth positions for a gentle warm-up.

>> Add torso curves or side bends if you want more expressive movement.

Technical Foundations

In this section, I define the technical terms that make up the foundation of every move in a Barre workout. You'll hear these terms used throughout this book and in many Barre classes, often as quick cues from an instructor while you are moving. Understanding what they mean helps you respond more confidently in the moment and get more out of each exercise.

Isolation

This technique helps you move one body part at a time so that you can build precision, control, and a stronger mind–body awareness.

What it is

Isolation is a movement technique that involves moving one part of your body independently from the others.

Why it matters

It improves your coordination, core engagement, and overall control.

How to do it

The isolation technique breaks down into three focused steps to help you gain control:

1. Stabilize your entire body except for the moving area.
2. Move that area using small, precise movements.
3. Keep your breath easy.

Do's and don'ts

» Do move slowly at first.

» Don't shift your hips or shoulders to compensate.

Variations

» Try rib isolations by gently moving your rib cage forward and back or side to side while keeping your hips and shoulders still. The movement is small and controlled, as if your ribs are gliding.

» Use hip isolations by subtly shifting or tilting your pelvis while keeping your upper body steady. Think of moving your hips independently without leaning, twisting, or letting your ribs join in.

Flexion

Flexion is a general movement term that describes bending or shortening at a joint. It can apply to many parts of your body, including your spine, hips, knees, arms, hands, and feet. In Barre, flexion is used to build strength, control, and awareness through precise, intentional movement.

What it is

Flexion occurs when you decrease the angle at a joint or gently round a part of the body. You are in flexion when you:

» Round your spine into a C-curve

» Bend your knees in a plié

» Draw your elbow or knee toward your body

» Pull your toes back toward your shin

Why it matters

Flexion strengthens muscles in their shortened position and helps stabilize your joints. Practicing flexion improves control, supports healthy movement patterns, and creates balance when paired with extension.

How to do it

The following steps outline flexion at the ankle, one example of flexion that you'll often see in a Barre workout:

1. Bend at the ankle so that your toes move toward your shin.

2. Keep the movement active rather than relaxed.

3. Maintain length through the rest of your body as you hold the position.

Do's and don'ts

» Do move with control and intention.

» Do keep the rest of your body aligned and supported.

» Do breathe steadily as you hold or repeat the movement.

» Don't force the range of motion.

» Don't collapse or grip through surrounding muscles.

Variations

» Alternate between flexion and extension to build balanced strength.

» Hold a flexed position longer to increase muscular engagement.

» Combine flexion with small pulses for added challenge.

Extension

Extension is a general movement term that describes straightening or lengthening at a joint. It can apply to many parts of your body, including your spine, hips, knees, arms, hands, and feet. In Barre, extension helps improve posture, mobility, and strength through long, open shapes.

What it is

Extension occurs when you increase the angle at a joint or lengthen part of the body. You are in extension when you:

» Lengthen your spine to stand tall

» Straighten your knees or elbows

>> Reach your arm or leg away from your body

>> Point your toes away from your shin

Why it matters

Extension strengthens muscles in their lengthened position and supports healthy alignment. Practicing extension improves posture, increases range of motion, and helps balance the strength built through flexion.

How to do it

The following steps outline extension at the ankle, which you'll often see in a Barre workout:

1. Lengthen at the ankle so that your toes point away from your shin.

2. Reach through the ball of your foot while keeping the leg active.

3. Maintain support through the rest of your body as you hold the position.

Do's and don'ts

>> Do lengthen through the joint rather than forcing it.

>> Do stay connected through your core and supporting muscles.

>> Do breathe steadily as you hold or repeat the movement.

>> Don't lock or hyperextend the joint.

>> Don't collapse into the movement without control.

Variations

>> Alternate between extension and flexion to build balanced strength.

>> Hold an extended position longer to increase muscular engagement.

>> Add small pulses or lifts to challenge control and endurance.

Flexibility

This essential physical quality helps you move through classical lines with ease while reducing the risk of injury.

What it is

Flexibility refers to the range of motion through your joints and muscles.

Why it matters

It supports healthy movement patterns and classical lines.

How to do it

Improving flexibility follows a few gentle rules to help your body open safely:

- **»** Warm up before you stretch.
- **»** Use dynamic stretches to prepare your body.
- **»** Hold controlled stretches to deepen mobility.

Do's and don'ts

- **»** Do stay consistent.
- **»** Don't force or bounce into a stretch.

Variations

- **»** Try active flexibility drills to build strength with mobility.
- **»** Use passive stretches when you want a deeper release.

ACTIVE FLEXIBILITY DRILLS

Active flexibility drills improve your range of motion by asking your muscles to work while you stretch. Instead of relaxing into a position and holding it, you actively control the movement in and out of the stretch.

Two simple examples you may encounter in a Barre workout include slowly lifting and lowering a straight leg while keeping the torso stable, or moving in and out of a controlled lunge while maintaining alignment. In both cases, your muscles stay engaged as you explore your range of motion, rather than relying on gravity alone.

Contraction

This expressive modern dance movement strengthens your core while adding shape and contrast to classical ballet movements.

What it is

A movement where your torso rounds inward from your center.

Why it matters

Contraction strengthens your core and improves expressive control.

How to do it

This movement unfolds in three steps to help you find depth and control:

1. Sit or stand tall.
2. Pull your abs toward your spine.
3. Round your torso gently.

Do's and don'ts

>> Do keep your shoulders relaxed.

>> Don't strain your neck.

Variations

>> Try seated contractions if you want more stability.

>> Use standing contractions to challenge your balance and control.

Classical Movements

In this section, you discover the classical ballet movements that have been cleverly adapted for Barre. These are the moving parts of ballet rather than the still poses. Think legs lifting, arms extending, and bodies controlling motion rather than holding that picture-perfect shape. If you have ever watched a ballet and thought, "Whoa, that looks beautiful and impossible," you have already seen these movements in action.

In Barre, these classical movements become challenging and targeted because of how they are performed. You repeat them, slow them down, and hold them. The muscles stay switched on, and your balance gets tested.

Plié

This essential ballet bend strengthens your legs, mobilizes your hips, and sets you up with clean alignment for almost every barre movement.

What it is

A plié is a classical ballet bend of the knees that maintains turnout and alignment.

Why it matters

It strengthens your legs, warms your joints, and supports proper posture for movement.

How to do it

Performing a plié involves a clear sequence to help you bend and rise with control:

1. Stand in first or second position.

2. Bend your knees over your toes while keeping your spine tall (Figure 5-5).

3. Press evenly through your feet to return to standing.

Do's and don'ts

» Do keep your heels grounded in demi-plié.

» Don't stick your seat out or collapse your arches.

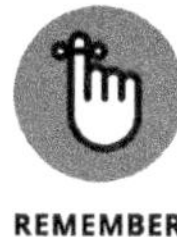
REMEMBER

A *demi-plié* refers to a small, subtle bend of the knees while keeping your heels on the floor. It is used throughout Barre to build leg strength, improve alignment, and protect the knees and ankles. Even though the movement is small, it plays a big role in helping your body move smoothly and safely.

Variations

» Try a deeper plié in second position to increase hip mobility.

» Add a relevé after your plié to build strength and balance.

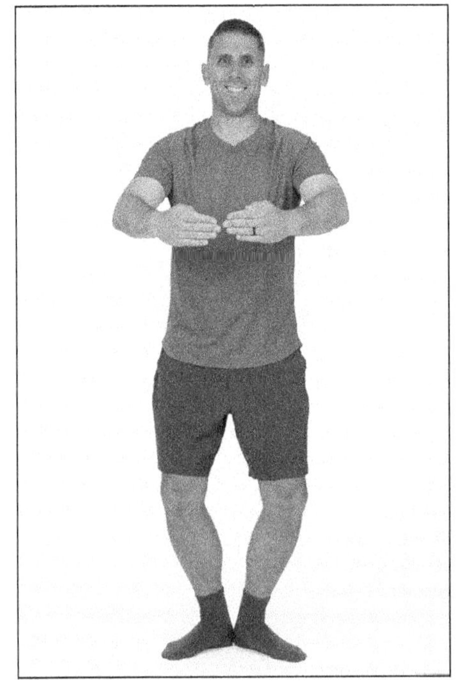

Tendu

This classical ballet slide or stretch of the foot teaches you to lengthen and articulate your legs and feet with precision and control.

What it is

A tendu is a stretch of your working foot along the floor to a fully extended point through your toes.

Why it matters

It builds strong feet, turnout awareness, and clean leg lines.

How to do it

This movement unfolds in three steps that help you articulate your feet:

1. Begin in first or fifth position.

2. Brush your foot along the floor until it is fully extended (Figure 5-6).

3. Close with control back to your starting position.

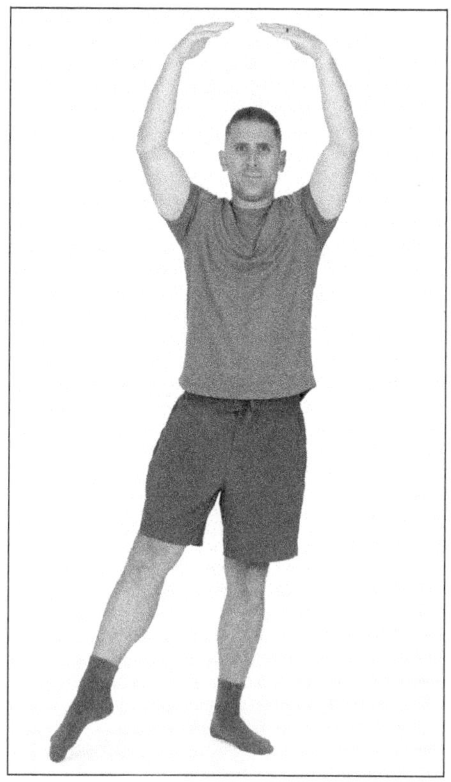

Do's and don'ts

>> Do keep your standing leg tall and stable.

>> Don't lift your working foot off the floor.

Variations

>> Try to explore different directions.

>> Add arm movements to improve coordination and balance.

Relevé

This lifted ballet position helps you develop balance, ankle strength, and clean alignment for elegant movement.

What it is

A relevé is a ballet position that is performed by rising onto the balls of your feet while maintaining a tall posture.

Why it matters

It improves your balance, strengthens your calves, and refines ankle control.

How to do it

This movement involves three steps to help you rise smoothly and safely:

1. Press through the balls of your feet.

2. Lift your heels with strong posture.

3. Lower with control (see Figures 5-7 and 5-8).

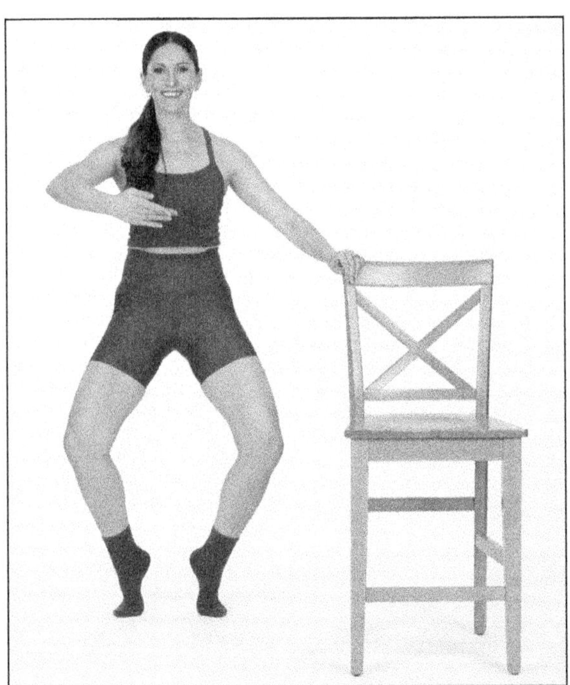

FIGURE 5-7: From your choice of starting position, press through the balls of your feet.

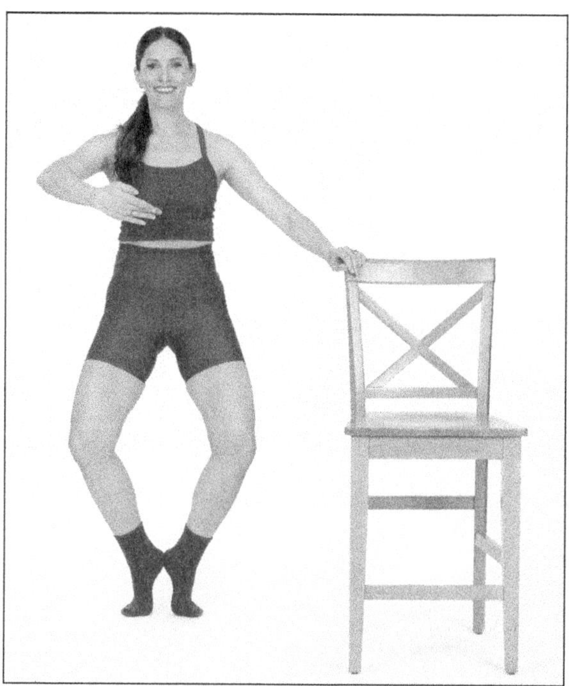

Do's and don'ts

>> Do keep your ankles aligned.

>> Don't roll onto the outer edges of your feet.

>> Don't be tempted to pulse; you never pulse a relevé!

Variation

Try a parallel relevé for stability or a turned-out relevé for classical technique.

Passé

Another lifted ballet position, the passé challenges your balance while helping you develop hip mobility and turnout control.

What it is

Meaning "passed" in French, a passé is a ballet position where your working foot lifts to touch your opposite knee.

Why it matters

It trains balance, turnout, and precise leg placement.

How to do it

This position builds through three steps to help you find balance and lift with your feet in a parallel or turnout position.

1. Stand tall in a parallel or turnout position.

2. Slide your foot up your standing leg to your knee (Figure 5-9).

3. Hold the position while keeping your hips square.

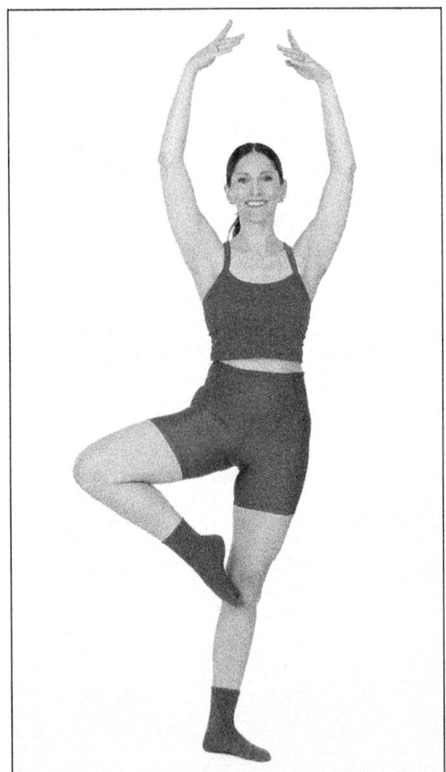

Do's and don'ts

>> Do keep your lifted knee pointing forward.

>> Don't tilt your pelvis.

Variations

>> Try doing a passé in parallel by keeping your standing foot facing forward rather than turned out. This reduces reliance on turnout and helps you focus on balance, alignment, and core stability. Working in parallel can feel more grounded and is a great option if you are building strength, managing knee or hip sensitivity, or simply want to refine control before adding rotation.

>> Use a turned-out passé by softly rotating your working leg outward from the hip while maintaining balance on your standing leg. This variation increases the challenge by asking your hips and deep stabilizing muscles to work harder.

Développé

This unfolding ballet movement helps you build strength, control, and flexibility as your leg extends into a long, clean line.

What it is

A développé is a smooth, gradual unfolding of your working leg into full extension.

Why it matters

It strengthens your hips, improves control, and develops long leg lines.

How to do it

Performing a développé breaks down into three steps that help you extend smoothly:

1. Draw your foot up to passé.

2. Extend your leg outward with control.

3. Lower with precision.

Do's and don'ts

>> Do keep your standing leg strong.

>> Don't lift your hip on the working side.

Variations

Perform it slowly to build strength or more quickly for coordination.

Devant, à la seconde, and derrière

These three classical ballet directions describe where your working leg extends in relation to your body: to the front, the side, or the back.

What it is

>> *Devant* means your working leg moves to the front of your body.

>> *À la seconde* means your working leg moves out to the side.

>> *Derrière* means your working leg moves to the back.

Why it matters

They help you develop clean lines, awareness of space, and correct pathways. These directions help teach your body how to move a limb through space with control, rather than just lifting it anywhere it feels easiest. In Barre, "correct pathways" refers to moving your leg along a clear, intentional line while keeping your torso stable and aligned. Over time, learning these pathways makes your movements feel smoother, stronger, and more confident. Here, your working leg extends to the front, side, or back, while maintaining strong posture and turnout.

How to do it

These directions build through simple placements that help you extend with clarity:

1. Begin in first or fifth position.

2. Extend your leg forward (devant), sideward (à la seconde), or backward (derrière).

3. Maintain your posture and hip alignment.

Do's and don'ts

» Do keep your weight centered over your standing leg.

» Don't tilt your pelvis.

Variations

» Experiment by exploring range and speed.

» Add arm positions to practice coordination.

Classical Ballet Poses

A classical ballet pose is a moment in movement, where the body briefly settles into a clear, intentional shape before transitioning to the next action. Unlike a classical position, which is often a starting or standing setup, a pose is usually the endpoint of a movement. It is where balance, alignment, and control come together.

In Barre, these poses often appear at the finish of a lift, extension, or balance exercise. You are not meant to hold them forever or perform them perfectly. Instead, they give your body a clear goal, helping you organize your muscles, refine coordination, and build confidence in your movement. Oh, and they're fun to do!

Attitude

This classic ballet pose challenges your balance and strength while helping you develop lifted, elegant leg lines.

What it is

A classical ballet attitude is a graceful pose where your working leg lifts with a gently bent knee.

Why it matters

It builds turnout, balance, hip strength, and control.

How to do it

The attitude pose builds through three steps to help you balance and lift with control:

1. Stand tall with your weight centered.

2. Lift your working leg forward, to the side, or back with a soft bend in your knee (Figure 5-10).

3. Maintain square hips and a lifted posture.

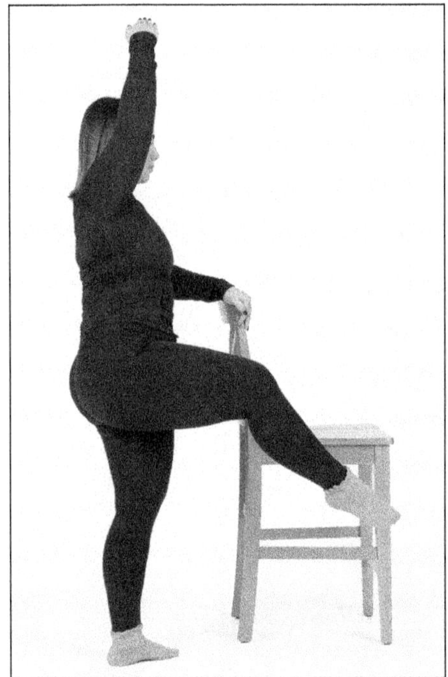

FIGURE 5-10: Maintain a lifted posture as you lift your working leg forward, to the side, or back with a soft bend in your knee.

Do's and don'ts

» Do lengthen through your spine.

» Don't arch your lower back or twist your hips.

Variations

» Try performing an attitude devant pose to strengthen your hip flexors.

» Use attitude derrière to activate your glutes and back body.

» Practice attitude à la seconde to challenge side stability.

Arabesque

This iconic ballet shape strengthens your back body while helping you create long, lifted, elegant lines.

What it is

An arabesque is a fundamental ballet pose where your leg lifts straight behind you (and looks incredibly graceful), with your arms outstretched in first, second, or third positions (or with one hand on your barre if needed).

Why it matters

It builds back strength, balance, turnout, and long leg lines.

How to do it

Performing an arabesque involves three steps to help you lift and lengthen with control:

1. Stand tall with your core engaged.

2. Lift your back leg straight behind you, point your toes while keeping your hips square. Your arms should be in first, second, or third position, and held out long and graceful with shaped hands. Hold onto a barre or yoga stick for extra support.

3. Reach forward through your upper body to lengthen your line (Figure 5-11).

Do's and don'ts

» Do keep your hips even.

» Don't sway your lower back or crunch your shoulders.

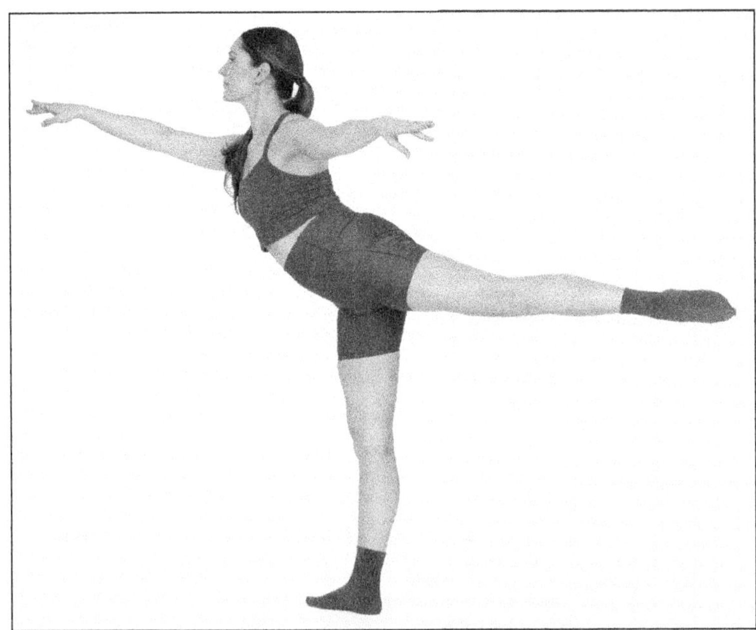

Variations

>> Try a low arabesque to work on alignment.

>> Raise your leg higher to increase strength and flexibility.

>> Add arm variations, such as both arms in high fifth or out to second position, to explore balance and artistry.

Penché

This dramatic ballet tilt helps you develop strength, flexibility, and balance while creating a beautifully long line.

What it is

A penché is a classical ballet pose where your torso tilts forward as your working leg lifts behind you.

Why it matters

Leaning forward builds hamstring flexibility, back strength, turnout control, and balance.

How to do it

Performing a penché involves **three steps** to help you tilt forward with stability and control:

1. Begin in an arabesque.

2. Slowly tilt your torso forward while lifting your back leg.

3. Keep your hips square as your leg and torso counterbalance.

Do's and don'ts

» Do reach long through both legs.

» Don't open your hips or bend your standing knee.

Variations

» Practice performing a supported penché by placing your hands on a barre for stability.

» Try small penché tilts to build confidence before going deeper.

» Add arm variations to challenge your balance.

Dynamic Movements and Training Concepts

Dynamic movements are exercises where the body moves through a range of motion with control and intention, rather than holding a single position. In Barre, these often include power kicks, active stretches, and controlled squats that ask muscles to lengthen and strengthen at the same time. The movement is purposeful and precise.

These dynamic exercises play an outsized role in Barre because they help build strength, coordination, and mobility together. They train your muscles to respond efficiently as you move, which supports balance, joint health, and overall athletic conditioning. Dynamic movement also helps warm the body thoroughly, preparing muscles and connective tissue for more sustained or challenging work later in the workout.

Battement

This powerful ballet kick strengthens your legs while helping you develop speed, control, and clean classical lines.

What it is

A battement in a Barre workout is a swift extension of your working leg that lifts upward from the hip.

Why it matters

Battement builds strength, flexibility, and dynamic control in your hips and legs.

How to do it

This movement builds through three steps that help you kick with power and control:

1. Stand tall with your core engaged.

2. Brush your working leg through a tendu stretch or dégagé.

3. Lift your leg to a controlled height and lower with precision (Figure 5-12).

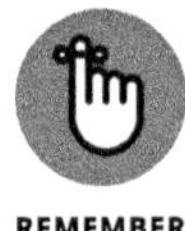

A dégagé is a small, quick extension of the leg where the foot lightly brushes off the floor and returns with control. Unlike a larger kick, the movement stays low and precise. In Barre, dégagé is often used to warm up the legs and refine control before bigger movements.

Do's and don'ts

>> Do keep your hips square.

>> Don't swing your leg or arch your back.

Variations

>> Try battement devant, à la seconde, and derrière to build full-range strength.

>> Use smaller kicks to refine control or higher kicks to challenge flexibility.

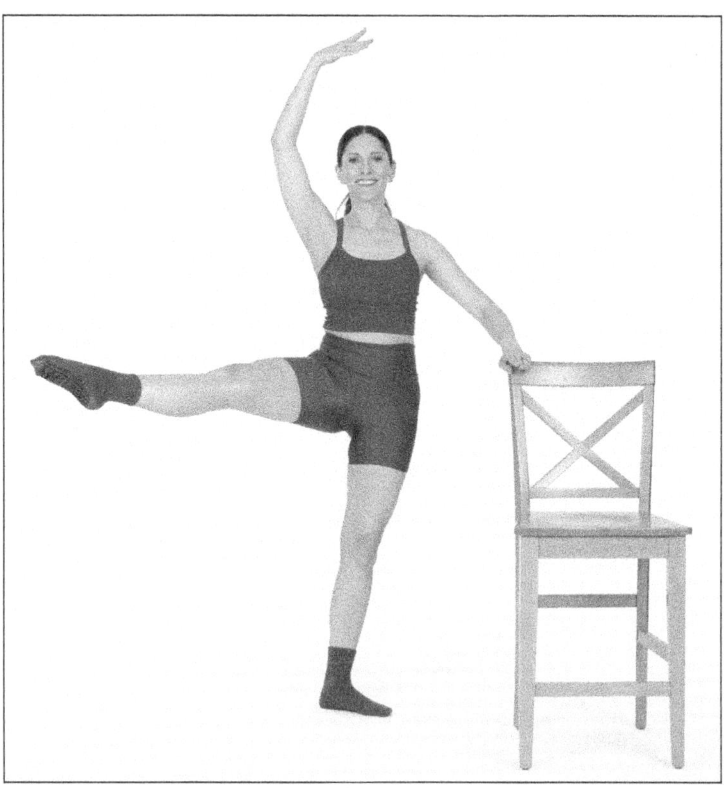

Pivot

This turning movement helps you develop coordination, alignment, and directional changes used throughout Barre and dance combinations.

What it is

A pivot is a controlled turn that rotates your body around your feet.

Why it matters

It improves coordination, balance, and comfort when moving through different directions.

How to do it

Performing a pivot follows clear steps that help you rotate with confidence:

1. Begin in a parallel stance.
2. Step forward, shifting your weight to the front foot.
3. Rotate your body in one smooth motion, foot brushing the floor, keeping your hips aligned.

Do's and don'ts

» Do keep your core strong.

» Don't twist your knees or lose alignment.

Variations

» Try half pivots to practice control.

» Add arm movements to challenge coordination.

Curtsy

This elegant lowering movement strengthens your legs and glutes while improving balance and coordination.

What it is

A curtsy is a crossed-leg bend where one leg steps behind the other as you lower your body.

Why it matters

It works your inner thighs, outer hips, and stabilizers while challenging balance.

How to do it

To curtsy, follow these steps to lower and rise smoothly:

1. With your hands on your hips, low rounded arms, or open to the second position, step one leg behind the other.
2. Bend both knees while keeping your chest lifted (Figure 5-13).
3. Press through your front foot to return to standing.

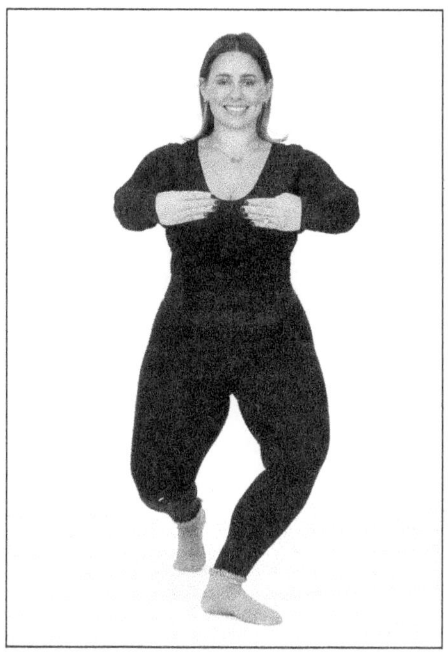

Do's and don'ts

» Do keep your hips facing forward.

» Don't collapse your chest or roll your knees inward.

Variations

» Take a deeper curtsy to challenge your glutes.

» Add a side leg lift to increase balance work.

Challenge zone

This training concept from my Xtend Method helps you build strength, endurance, and confidence by working at an intensity that feels effortful but achievable. The zone is completely personal to your ability and can, of course, change over time. It's a way to be physically aware and accountable, and asks the question: Can you safely push yourself a little more? If the answer is yes, you've found your challenge zone!

What it is

The challenge zone is a focused effort level where you work just outside what feels comfortable.

Why it matters

It helps you gain strength, improve stamina, and make consistent progress.

How to do it

To safely and effectively push your boundaries by working in your challenge zone, follow these guidelines:

1. Choose an exercise you know well.
2. Increase your range, tempo, or repetitions slightly.
3. Maintain control without losing form.

Do's and don'ts

» Do really listen to your body.

» Don't sacrifice form in pursuit of intensity.

Variations

» Hold the exercises longer to build endurance.

» Add light weights or pulses to increase the challenge.

2

Meet Me at the Barre: Component Exercises

Walk through a warm-up sequence to evenly activate your muscles, safely elevate your heart rate, and prepare your body for what's ahead.

Work your upper body by flowing through a nonstop series that will help you sculpt muscle, improve postural strength and alignment, and feel strong and graceful.

Discover the classic moves at the heart of a Barre workout that are designed to target the lower body.

Strengthen your core with a workout that targets your powerhouse muscles with small, precise movements.

Flow through a nonstop series of lower-body exercises that fire up your glutes, hips, and thighs.

Finish strong with active stretches and two cool-down moments to help you recenter and close your Barre session.

Chapter 6

Warming Up

Every Barre workout starts with a targeted warm-up to evenly activate your muscles, safely elevate your heart rate, and prepare your body for what's ahead through a variety of planes of movement. This chapter walks you through a go-to warm-up sequence that focuses on postural strength and alignment with variations and repetitions, and sets your intention with positive, upbeat energy.

Exercises in This Chapter

The exercises in this chapter include the following:

» Knee-Lift Series

» Plié Tendu

» First-Position Lunge Back

» Side Reach

» Curtsy Pliés

For each exercise, I first help you prepare, and then I provide detailed steps for each one, followed by do's and don'ts to keep in mind as you practice. Finally, each section ends with ideas for variation.

Knee-Lift Series

This knee-lift exercise, which incorporates a series of five simple arm movements, focuses on your hamstrings and quadriceps to strengthen hip and knee extensors, warm up large muscle groups, and develop lower-body alignment and pelvic lumbar stabilization. Do 8 repetitions (up to 2 sets) at each stage.

Getting set

Stand with your feet hip-width apart in a parallel stance, and keep your arms relaxed and down by your sides.

The movement

Work through each of the following five stages while doing the following movement:

Lift one leg off the floor with a slight bend in your knee. Replace it on the floor, as shown in Figure 6-1. Repeat on your other leg.

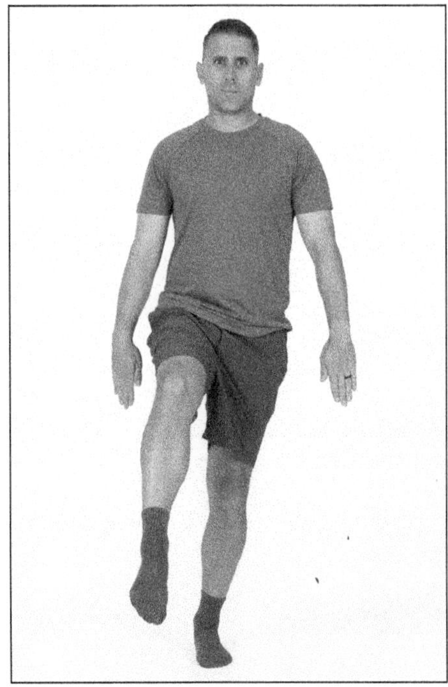

FIGURE 6-1:
Stand with your feet hip-width apart and raise each knee in turn throughout this warm-up.

1. **Begin with oppositional arms.**

    a. Swing your arms in opposition to your legs. Do a controlled swing, reaching to the sky and to the floor.

    b. Do 8 repetitions (up to 2 sets).

2. **Flow into a forward press.**

    a. Press your arms (palms forward) to the front of your body, in line with your chest.

    b. Draw your arms back wide with your hands to your shoulders and your elbows behind your body.

    c. Do 8 repetitions (up to 2 sets).

3. **Flow into a side press.**

    a. Press your arms (palms out) to the side of your body at shoulder height.

    b. Do 8 repetitions (up to 2 sets).

4. **Flow into an upward press.**

    a. Extend your arms overhead (palms up). Draw your arms back in with your hands to your shoulders. Your elbows come down to the side of your ribcage.

    b. Do 8 repetitions (up to 2 sets).

5. **Flow into rotation.**

    a. Open your arms to your side with a 90-degree bend (think "goalpost"). Rotate from your torso, twist your upper body toward your lifted leg, and dip your elbows down, as shown in Figure 6-2.

    b. Do 8 repetitions (up to 2 sets).

Finish with your feet in first position for lunge backs, or open to second position.

Do's and don'ts

» Do articulate foot placement; think: "toe, ball, heel."

» Do maintain a long neutral spine.

» Do keep your abdominals engaged.

» Do open your chest and relax your shoulders.

» Don't bring your chest to your leg; instead, bring your thigh toward your chest.

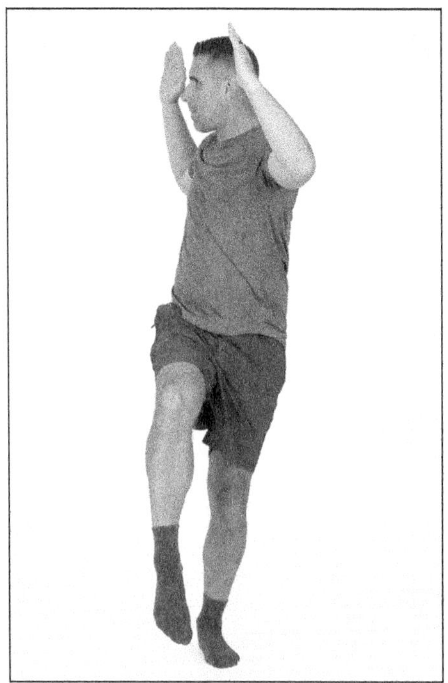

Variations

>> Modify by decreasing the range of motion or the number of repetitions.

>> Progress by increasing the range of motion and number of repetitions.
To further advance, add light arm weights.

Plié Tendu

This classic Barre move focuses on your hamstrings, quadriceps, and gluteus muscles to strengthen hip and knee extensors, warm up large muscle groups, and develop pelvic lumbar stabilization. Do 8 repetitions for each set and up to 4 sets.

Getting set

Stand tall in the center of the floor. Open your arms and legs to the second position, as shown in Figure 6-3.

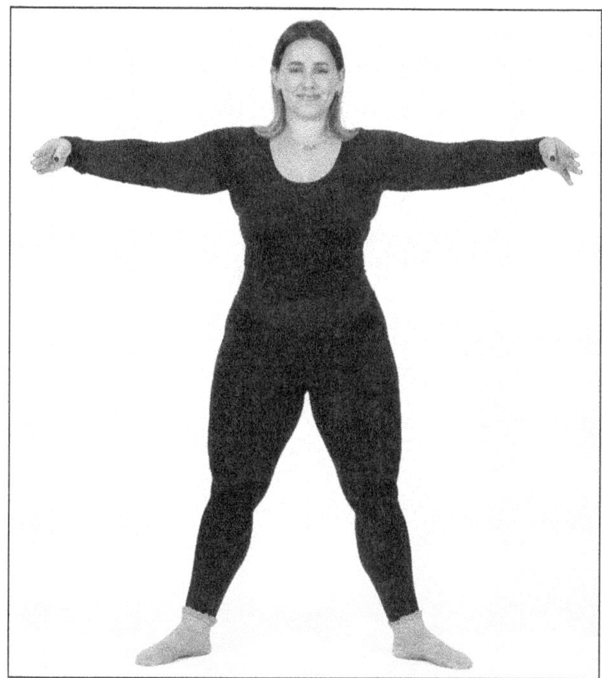

The movement

The movement involves three stages:

1. **Bend the knees to plié.**

   a. Draw your arms to the low fifth position, holding them in a graceful oval shape.

   b. Finish with your hands at your waist.

2. **Maintaining your plié, transition your weight to your right foot.**

   a. Extend both legs and point your left foot to the floor.

   b. Open your arms to second position (Figure 6-4).

3. **Plié and repeat on the other side.**

Move slowly enough to really feel the weight shift from one foot to the other. If you rush the transition, you miss the stabilizing work in the hips and core that makes this exercise so effective.

Increase the range of motion of your arms by drawing your arms from the low fifth position in plié to a high V position as your legs extend.

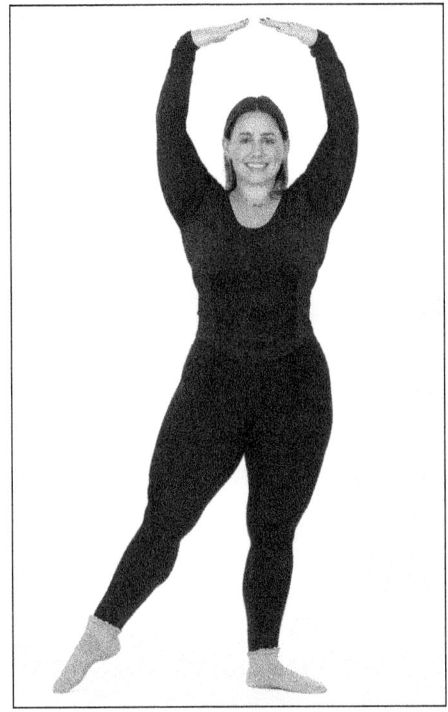

Finish by holding in second position.

Do's and don'ts

>> Do draw energy through your supporting heel (activating the glutes to raise your body).

>> Do focus on your core control when you lower and lift.

>> Do keep your shoulders down and a neutral spine.

>> Do lengthen through your quads on tendu.

Variations

>> Modify by keeping your arms in second position or below your shoulders.

>> Progress with a battement, increase the depth of your plié, and/or add light arm weights.

First-Position Lunge Back

This lunge-back exercise, starting in first position, involves three stages that focus on your hip extensors, gluteus muscles, and core to lengthen the hip adductors and develop pelvic lumbar stabilization through balance. Do 8 to 16 repetitions for each set (up to 2 sets).

Getting set

Stand with your feet and hands in first position, as shown in Figure 6-5.

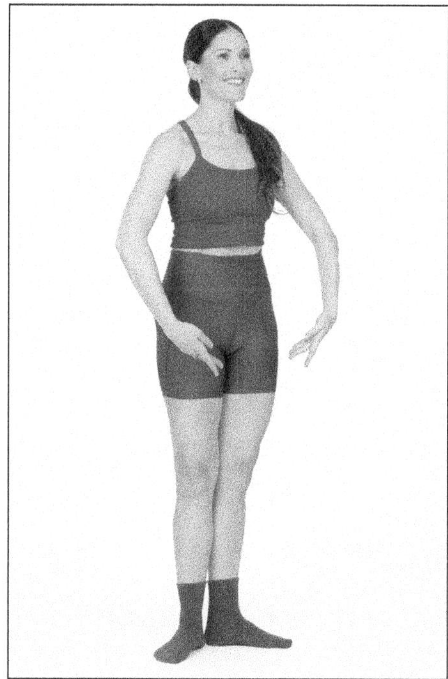

The movement

Work through each of the following three stages while doing the following movement:

Bend your left leg as you slide your right leg straight back, your arms lifting to high fifth position (creating a long line lunge), as shown in Figure 6-6. Return to the start position. Repeat on the same leg or the other side.

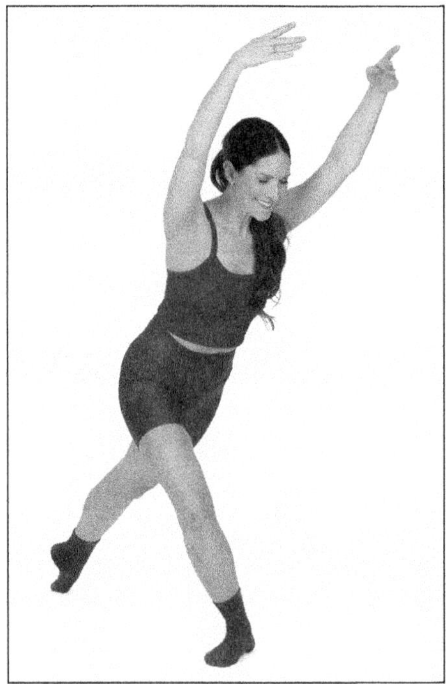

1. **Hold your leg in a lunge position and pulse back upward.**

   Do 8 to 16 repetitions for each set (up to 2 sets).

2. **Then, hold your leg in lunge position and pulse the front leg down.**

   Do 8 to 16 repetitions for each set (up to 2 sets).

3. **Finally, do a combination, pulse back leg up and front leg down.**

   Do 8 to 16 repetitions for each set (up to 2 sets).

Finish by stepping to second position or curtsy your working leg back.

Do's and don'ts

» Do maintain a long spine.

» Do keep your abdominals engaged.

» Do keep your hips and shoulders square.

» Do keep your hips forward and your thigh back to engage the glutes.

Variations

» Modify by decreasing the range of motion for beginners or those with injuries.

» Progress by adding light arm weights.

Side Reach

This exercise, which begins with a wide-leg stance in the second position, has two main components — Side Reach 1 and Side Reach 2 — with variations. The Side Reach focuses on your abdominals, especially your obliques, warming up your core muscles while incorporating a full-body movement. Do 8 repetitions for each set.

Getting set

Standing center floor, open your legs to a wide second position with natural turn-out and get ready to plié.

The movement

The movement involves three stages:

1. **Begin with side reach 1.**

   a. Hold your right arm to the side of your body in a goalpost position with your left hand on your hip, and plié.

   b. Laterally flex your spine to the left, drawing the left base of your ribs to your left hip, as your right arm lengthens (Figure 6-7).

   c. Return to the start position.

   d. Repeat.

   e. Repeat the full sequence on the other side.

   f. Do 8 repetitions.

2. **Flow into side reach with elbow to hip.**

   a. With your right elbow to your right hip, increase your range of motion by flexing your spine laterally in both directions, cinching the waistline (Figure 6-8).

   b. Repeat on the left side.

   c. Do 8 repetitions (up to 2 sets).

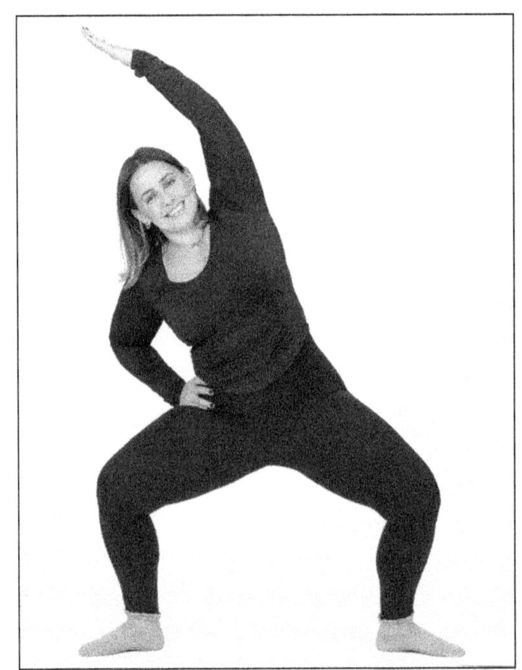

FIGURE 6-7:
In a plié, laterally
flex your spine
and lengthen the
opposite arm.

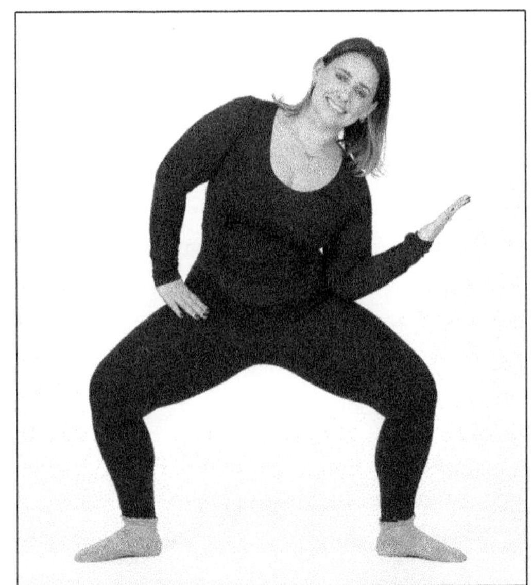

FIGURE 6-8:
In a plié, tuck
your right elbow
into your right
hip, and reach to
both sides
alternately.

3. **Flow into side reach 2.**

TIP

   a. Plié in second position, laterally flex your spine, reaching your right arm to the high fifth position and your left arm to the low fifth position.

   As you reach into high fifth and low fifth, think about lifting up and over rather than collapsing sideways. Keeping length through both sides of your waist helps the obliques work without squishing the spine.

   b. Lift back up and tendu your left leg with your arms in second position.

   c. Repeat.

   d. Repeat the full sequence on the other side.

   e. Do 8 repetitions (up to 2 sets).

Option 1: Side passé

Repeat stages 1, 2, and 3, replacing the tendu with a passé (see Chapter 5 for more on how to perform a passé). Do 8 repetitions (up to 2 sets).

Option 2: Side battement

Repeat stages 1, 2, and 3, replacing the passé with a battement (see Chapter 5 for more on how to perform a battement). Do 8 repetitions (up to 2 sets). Finish by holding the second position or stepping your leg behind to curtsy.

Do's and don'ts

>> Do perform movements in the frontal plane.

>> Do keep your lower body still, attempting a deep plié.

>> Do imagine a dowel across the trapezoids; keep your upper body lifted.

>> Do keep your hips square, abdominals in, and shoulders down.

Variations

>> Modify by reducing the range of motion.

>> Progress by adding light hand weights or a small ball for Side Reach 1.

Curtsy Pliés

This exercise, which starts with a wide-leg stance in second position, has two main components: The foundation curtsy and the advanced curtsy. Focusing on your hamstrings and quadriceps, curtsy pliés are great for developing body awareness while warming up large muscle groups. Do 8 to 16 repetitions for each position.

Getting set

Stand in a wide leg stance in the center of the floor, with your legs and arms open to second position (see Figure 6-3 earlier in this chapter).

The movement

The movement involves two components — the foundation curtsy and the advanced curtsy — with variations.

1. **Start with the foundation curtsy.**

   a. Step your right leg from second position to curtsy, closing your arms to first position (Figure 6-9).

   b. Open your legs and arms back to second position.

      Curtsy pulse: Hold curtsy with arms overhead in high fifth position and pulse.

      Arms: Hold a deep curtsy, reach arms up/down from low fifth position to high fifth position.

   c. Switch sides and repeat the entire series on your left leg.

   d. Do 8 to 16 repetitions for each position.

2. **Flow into an advanced curtsy.**

   a. Step your right leg from second position to a deeper curtsy, reaching your right arm toward the floor and extending your left arm on a high diagonal.

   b. Open your legs and arms back to second position.

      Tendu: Step your right foot to tendu as your arms open to second position.

      Passé: Lift your right leg up to passé as your arms open to second position.

   c. Do 8 to 16 repetitions for each position.

Finish by holding second position.

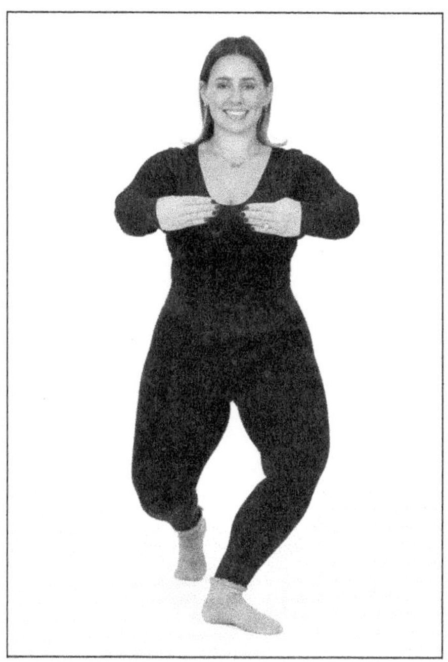

Do's and don'ts

>> Do keep your movements fluid and graceful.

>> Do keep your hips and shoulders square.

>> Do make sure you place your weight evenly on your supporting foot.

Variations

>> Modify by making your pliés very small, or performing no movement at all, and just holding the position.

>> Progress by increasing your range of motion and/or repetitions.

>> Progress further by lifting both hands off the barre to the high fifth position and maintaining balance.

Chapter **7**

Waking the Upper Body

This chapter focuses on waking up your upper-body muscles evenly with small, controlled movements that target your biceps, shoulders, chest, back, and triceps. With light to medium weights (or even none at all), and working in all planes of movement, you'll sculpt muscle, improve postural strength and alignment, and feel strong and graceful from the very first repetition. From here, you can easily upgrade to incorporate the lower body to create compound movement, activating even more muscle groups. No barre required.

Barre is wonderful for targeting specific muscles, even ones you didn't know you had! But compound movement, using two or more muscle groups and joint areas in harmony, is also a major Barre component.

TECHNICAL
STUFF

Exercises in This Chapter

The exercises in this chapter include the following:

» Bicep Curls

» 90-Degree Lifts

» Waltzing

» Arm Circles

>> Port de Bras Arms

>> Hug and Carriage

>> Swimming and Temperature

>> V-Press

>> Rowing and Puppet

>> Hinge Swing Fly Series

>> Curtsy Triceps

>> Triceps Lunges

For each exercise, I first help you prepare, and then I provide detailed steps for each one, followed by do's and don'ts to keep in mind as you practice. Finally, each section ends with ideas for variation.

To complete the exercises in this chapter, choose weights that allow you to move with control rather than momentum. If your shoulders creep up, your grip tightens, or your form slips, go lighter or drop the weights altogether. In Barre, precision always beats heaviness.

Bicep Curl

You'll need a set of light or medium hand weights for this exercise, which focuses on your biceps and deltoids to strengthen and sculpt your shoulders and arms. Hold the weights firmly in the crook of your thumb joint with your fingers outstretched and relaxed. I always encourage new clients to start with a light weight, even if they're confident of their strength, as this exercise can be more challenging than it seems; it really creeps up on you! There are nine key moves to flow through. Do 8 to 16 repetitions for each set.

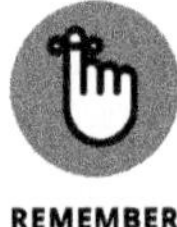

Make sure you keep your elbows and knees soft, shoulders down and relaxed, and your abdominals engaged throughout.

Getting set

Stand in the center of the floor in a parallel stance, feet hip-width apart, and with a slight bend in your knees. Holding your hand weights, lift your arms straight up to a horizontal position, slightly wider and lower than your shoulders, with your palms face up.

The movement

Flow through each of the following nine moves, keeping your muscles activated on both the up and down movements:

1. **Start with a single bicep curl.**

   a. Flex at the elbow, drawing your fingertips toward your shoulder.

   b. Slowly extend your arm back to the starting position.

   c. Repeat with your other arm.

   d. Do 8 to 16 repetitions for each set.

2. **Flow into double bicep curls.**

   a. Flex both your elbows at the same time, as in stage 1 and as shown in Figure 7-1.

   b. Extend both arms back to the starting position.

   c. Do 8 to 16 repetitions for each set.

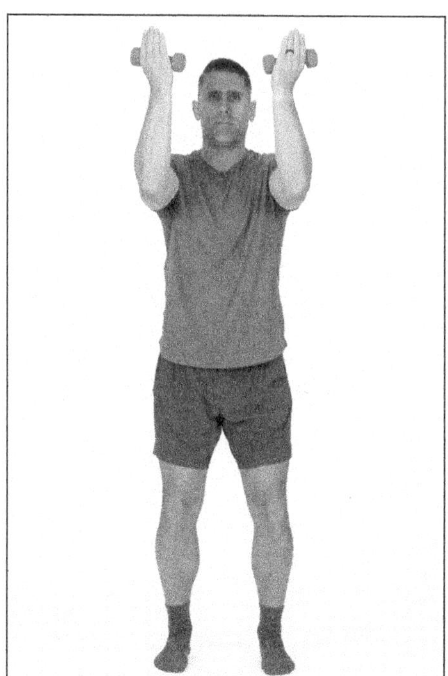

FIGURE 7-1: Flex both your elbows at the same time.

3. **Then, do alternating bicep curls.**

   a. Using both your arms, alternate your bicep curls simultaneously (Figure 7-2).

   b. Do 8 to 16 repetitions for each set.

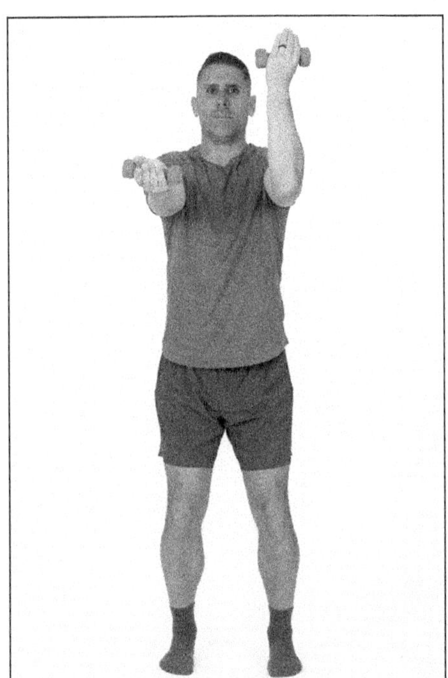

4. **Flow into mini bicep curls.**

   a. Flex both your elbows in slightly, then fully extend your arms out at the same time, slowly and mindfully.

   b. Do 8 to 16 repetitions for each set.

Take a quick moment to reset your shoulders, keeping them down and relaxed, and your abs activated.

TIP

5. **Do arm circles.**

   a. Hold your arms out horizontally and, with a relaxed but firm grip on your weights, draw small circles in the air (try for a 10-inch circumference).

   b. Change direction.

   c. Do 8 to 16 repetitions for each set.

6. **Flow into pulses.**

   a. With both arms held out horizontally in front of you and with a slight flex in your elbows, pulse your arms up a few inches.

   b. Do 8 to 16 repetitions for each set.

7. **Flow into the W/X movement.**

   a. Open your arms to the sides of your body with your elbows close to your waist in a W shape.

   b. Bring your arms in front of your body in an X position, keeping your elbows tucked into your waist (Figure 7-3).

   c. Open your arms back out to the sides of your body.

   d. Repeat, alternating the wrist on top.

   e. Do 8 to 16 repetitions for each set.

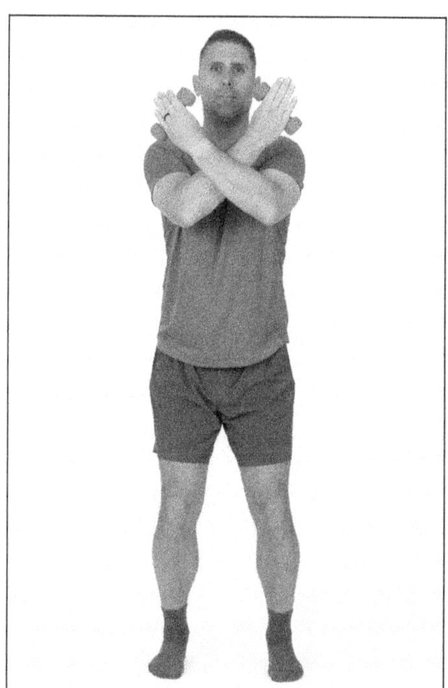

FIGURE 7-3: Flow into an X stance.

8. **Flow into a high and low fifth position.**

   a. Lift your arms to a high fifth "X" with your wrists crossed and your palms facing forward.

b. Open your arms to your sides and down to a low fifth position with your wrists crossed and your palms facing your body.

c. Repeat, alternating your front arm.

d. Do 8 to 16 repetitions for each set.

9. **Do the X-extend.**

a. Start with your forearms crossed in an "X" position, your humerus (upper arm) parallel with the floor.

b. Extend your arms in line with your shoulders (like train tracks) and flex back into an "X."

c. Hold the "X" and pulse up, raising your elbows a couple of inches.

d. Do 8 to 16 repetitions for each set.

Finish the series by comfortably extending your arms, ready for 90-degree lifts.

Work slowly and mindfully with resistance on both the upward and downward movements.

Do's and don'ts

» Do maintain soft knees and elbows throughout.

» Do keep your hips and shoulders square.

» Don't allow your shoulders to rise up and tense; keep them low and relaxed.

» Do keep your abdominals engaged.

Variations

» Modify by limiting your range of motion or using a lighter hand weight.

» Progress by increasing repetitions.

90-Degree Lifts

You'll need a set of light weights for this exercise, which, like the bicep curls, focuses on your biceps and deltoids to strengthen and sculpt your shoulders and arms. You'll flow through four stages with your arms at 90 degrees (right angle) and light weights in your hands held firmly in the crook of your thumb joint with your fingers extended and relaxed. Remember to keep your elbows and knees soft and your abdominals engaged. Do 8 to 16 repetitions and up to 4 sets.

Getting set

Stand in the center of the floor in a parallel stance, feet hip-width apart, a slight bend in your knees, your arms lifted in front of the body parallel to the floor like train tracks, and weights in hand, as shown in Figure 7-4.

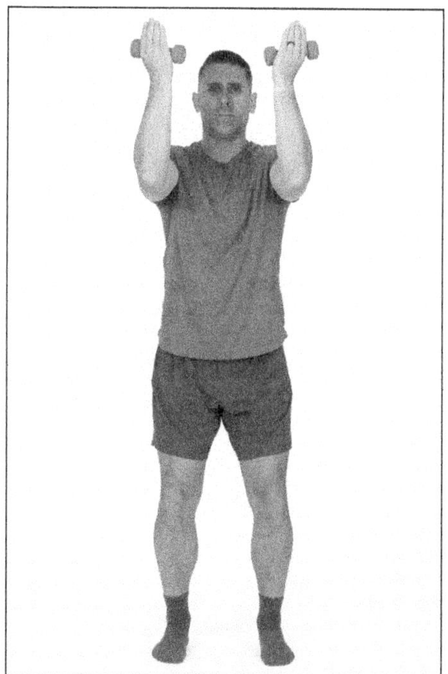

The movement

The movement involves four stages:

1. **Start with 90-degree lifts with extension (front).**

   a. From the starting position, flex your elbows to 90 degrees only, keeping your humerus (upper arm) parallel to the floor and your palms toward your face.

   b. Extend your arms back to the start position and repeat.

   c. Do 8 to 16 repetitions (up to 4 sets).

   Optional add-on: Add tiny pulses as you flex.

2. **Flow into 90-degree lifts with extension (side).**

   a. Start with your arms to your sides in a T shape with your palms facing up.

   b. Flex your elbows to 90 degrees only, keeping your upper arm parallel to the floor and your palms facing the sides of your face.

   c. Extend your arms back to the start position and repeat.

   d. Do 8 to 16 repetitions (up to 4 sets).

   Optional add-on: Add tiny pulses as you flex.

3. **Flow into 90-degree bend (open/close).**

   a. Start with your arms in a goalpost position or H-shape (Figure 7-5).

   b. Close your arms by bringing your elbows toward each other until they are in line with your shoulders, maintaining a 90-degree angle.

   c. Open your arms back to the starting position, with your palms facing in.

   d. Do 8 to 16 repetitions (up to 4 sets).

   Optional add-on: Add tiny pulses as you flex.

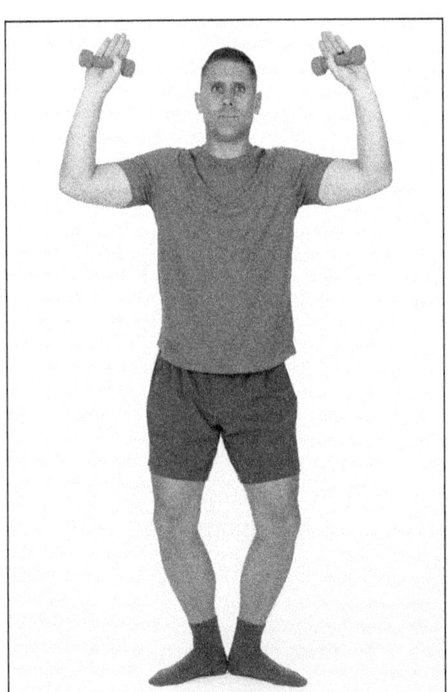

FIGURE 7-5: Start with your arms in an H-shape.

4. **Flow into a 90-degree bend (add up/down).**

   a. Repeat stage 3, the open/close series, adding a lift when the arms are in front of the body. (Think: "open the arms, close the arms, lift and lower.")

   b. Do 8 to 16 repetitions (up to 4 sets).

This lift is very small, just a couple of inches.

Finish by bringing the arms to high fifth position ready for waltzing.

Do's and don'ts

>> Do maintain soft knees and elbows.

>> Do maintain neutral shoulders while your arms are lifted.

>> Do deepen your abdominals as your arms close.

>> Don't just use gravity; remember to resist up and down.

>> Focus on your form: "how" not "how many."

Variations

>> Modify by limiting your range of motion.

>> Progress by using single-arm actions for any of the four series.

Waltzing

Inspired by the classic Viennese ballroom dance, you'll need a set of light weights for this exercise, which focuses on your medial deltoids and upper trapezius muscles to strengthen and define your shoulders and upper back. Weights should be held firmly in the crook of your thumb joint with your fingers extended and relaxed. You'll flow into four stages. Remember to keep your elbows and knees soft and your abdominals engaged. For any shoulder issues, check out the Variations. Do 8 to 16 repetitions for each set.

Getting set

Stand in the center of the floor, feet in the second position with heels together, your arms in a high V shape (think of a classic cheerleader stance), weights in hand, and palms facing outward, as shown in Figure 7-6.

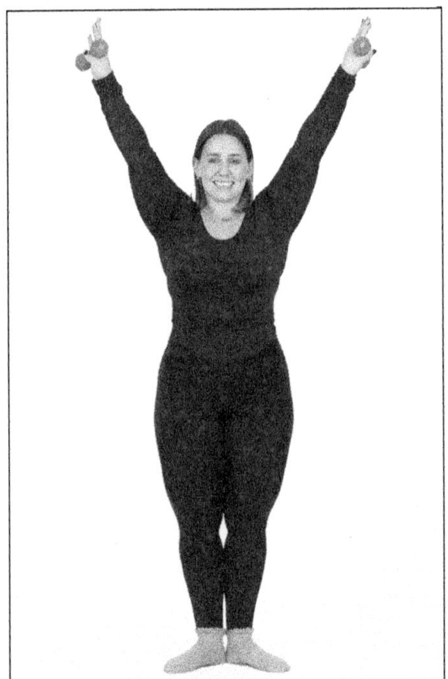

The movement

The movement involves three stages:

1. **Start with a high V sweep.**

   a. From your high V position with palms facing outward, sweep your arms to a high fifth position, the classic, graceful oval shape, with your palms facing inward, as shown in Figure 7-7.

   b. Sweep your arms back out to a V shape, palms facing outward again, and repeat.

   c. Do 8 to 16 repetitions for each set.

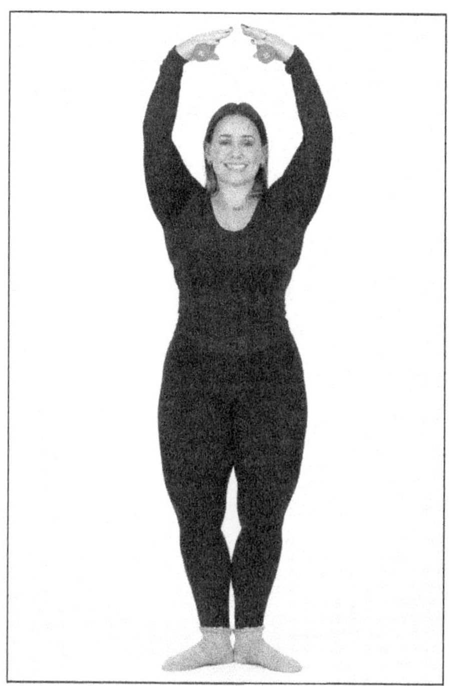

2. **Flow into biceps (double).**

   a. From your high V position, tap your fingers to your shoulders and back out to a V shape.

   b. Do 8 to 16 repetitions for each set.

3. **Flow into biceps (single).**

   a. Repeat the move in stage 2, but perform single-arm taps and/or alternate your arms, as shown in Figure 7-8.

   b. Do 8 to 16 repetitions for each set.

Finish by holding your balance and keeping your arms open to your sides.

Do's and don'ts

>> Do maintain shoulder stability when lifting your arms.

>> Do keep your abdominals engaged.

>> Do maintain soft knees and elbows.

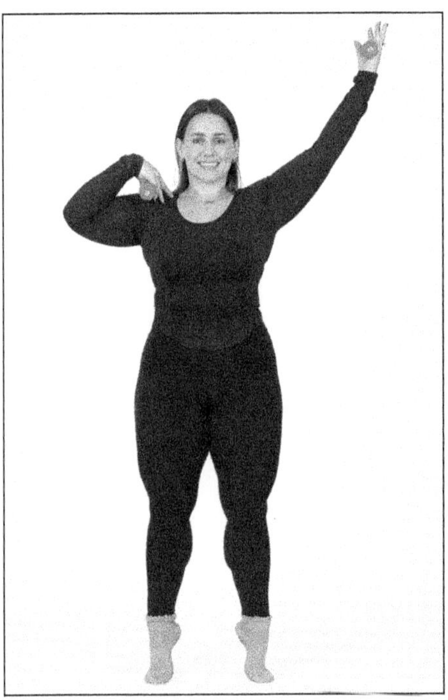

Variations

>> Modify by omitting the weights and/or limiting your range of motion (for shoulder issues, do not lift your arms above shoulder height).

>> Progress by performing a plié to relevé.

Arm Circles

This simple deltoid-focused exercise with light or medium hand weights strengthens and sculpts the front and middle shoulders. Weights should be held firmly in the crook of your thumb joint with your fingers extended and relaxed. Remember to keep your elbows and knees soft and your abdominals engaged. You'll flow into three stages, and stages 1 and 2 are particularly small, careful movements. For stage 3, if you have any shoulder issues, do not lift your arms above shoulder height. Do 8 to 16 repetitions for each set.

It's easy to just swing through stage 3 of this exercise. For a more targeted workout, move mindfully, keeping your muscles activated, and avoid using gravity.

Getting set

Stand in the center of the floor with your feet hip-distance apart or in second position and weights in hand.

The movement

The movement involves three stages:

1. **Start with arm circles (front).**

   a. Begin with your arms straight out in front of the body, parallel to the floor and in line with your shoulders, weights in hand, palms down or up (Figure 7-9).

   b. Begin to move your arms in small circles, within the frame of your shoulders. Really concentrate on the "up" of the movement.

   c. Repeat your arm circles in the reverse direction.

   d. Do 8 to 16 repetitions for each set.

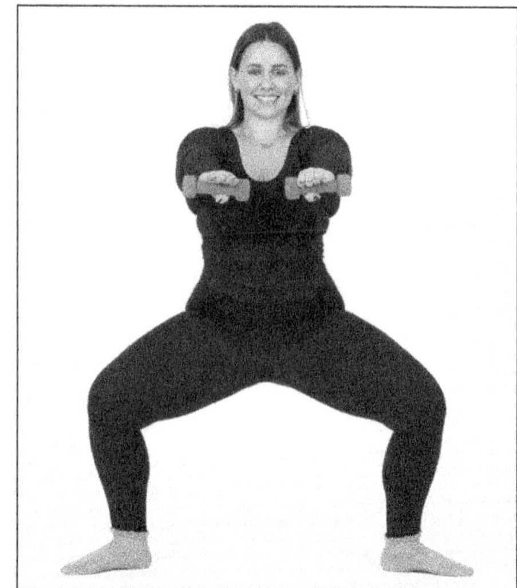

FIGURE 7-9: Begin with your arms straight out in front of your body, standing, or in a plié as shown here.

2. Flow into arm circles (side).

a. This is the same movement as in stage 1, but with your arms to the side, parallel with the floor, weights in hand, palms facing down or up (Figure 7-10).

b. Begin to move your arms in small circles, within the frame of your shoulders. As before, really concentrate on the "up" of the movement.

c. Repeat your arm circles in the reverse direction.

d. Do 8 to 16 repetitions for each set.

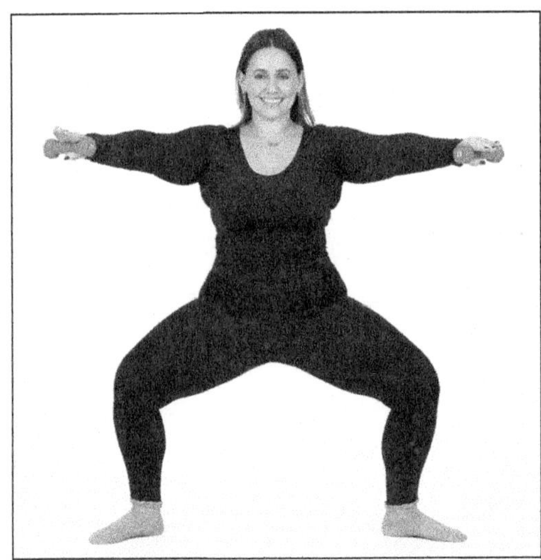

FIGURE 7-10: Reposition your arms to the side, standing or in a plié.

3. Flow into postural arm swings (right and left).

a. Begin with both your arms down and to the side of your body, palms facing in, weights in hand.

b. Lift your right arm straight up to the side of your head, vertical to the floor, as the left hand presses slightly behind your pelvis.

c. With control, sweep the arms to alternate positions.

d. Repeat on the other side, moving with precision and control.

e. Do 8 to 16 repetitions for each set.

Finish by extending your arms longer.

Do's and don'ts

» Do concentrate on your posture and flow of movement.

» Do keep your abdominals engaged.

» Do focus on your upper body stability, keeping your shoulders down and relaxed.

» Don't allow tension to creep into your head, neck, or shoulders.

Variations

» Modify by omitting the weights and/or limiting your range of motion (for shoulder issues, do not lift your arms above shoulder height).

» Progress by adding in lower-body options, including performing a plié to relevé.

Port de Bras Arms

This gorgeous-looking ballet move, meaning "carriage of the arms," is also a classic Barre component. It's with this exercise that you can channel your inner principal dancer with graceful, fluid motion: soft, rounded arms and lifted elbows, curved wrists, and relaxed fingers. With light hand weights tucked into the crook of your thumb joint, you'll activate your deltoids and pectoralis major to develop both trunk and scapula stabilization. Do 8 repetitions for each set.

Getting set

In the center of the floor, stand with your feet in first position with a soft bend in your knees. Place your arms in first position, with your elbows higher than your wrists (forming a soft, graceful oval as if you are holding a beach ball), and hold your light hand weights.

The movement

The movement involves three stages:

1. **Start with the single-arm hug series.**

   a. Open your arms to second position.

   b. Bring your right hand to first position and then back to second position.

   c. Repeat with your left hand.

   d. Do 8 repetitions with single arms.

2. **Flow into the double-arm hug series.**

   a. Move both arms together to first position and then back to second position.

   b. Repeat with double arms.

   c. Do 8 to 16 repetitions.

Alternatively, bring your right arm, and then your left arm, from first position back to second position.

3. **Flow into carriage of the arms (port de bras).**

   a. Begin with your arms in front of your body in first position.

   b. Draw your arms above your head in a high fifth position, then down to your sides in second position.

   c. Lower your arms down in front of your pelvis in a low fifth position.

   d. Do 4 repetitions in each direction.

Finish by pivoting your feet to parallel or open to second position.

Do's and don'ts

>> Do keep your abs in and up.

>> Do maintain soft knees.

>> Do move gracefully with control and resistance.

Variations

>> Modify by eliminating your weights.

>> Progress by adding battement.

Hug and Carriage

Drawing from classical ballet and incorporating the previous exercise, port de bras arms, this graceful exercise focuses on your deltoids and pectoralis major to strengthen and sculpt your chest and torso and develop torso and scapula stabilization. I also added a leg sequence to focus on your thighs and glutes. You'll need a set of light weights (tucked into the crook of your thumb joint with your fingers extended and relaxed), and you'll flow through three movements with different stages. Remember to keep your elbows and knees soft and your abs engaged. Do 8 repetitions for each set.

Getting set

Stand in the center of the floor with your feet in first position with a soft bend in your knees, weights in hand, and your arms in first position, as shown in Figure 7-11.

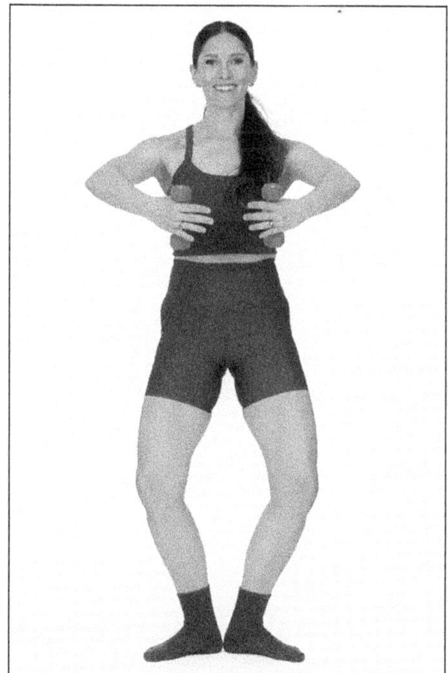

FIGURE 7-11: This is the starting position for hug and carriage.

The movement

The movement involves five stages:

1. **Start with the single-arm hug series.**

   a. With your muscles engaged, open your arms to second position.

   b. Bring your right hand to first position and then back to second position.

   c. Repeat with your left hand.

   d. Do 8 repetitions for each set.

2. **Flow into double arms.**

   a. Move both arms together to first position and then back to second position.

   b. Do 8 repetitions for each set.

3. **Flow into alternate arms.**

   a. Alternate bringing your right arm and then left arm from first position back to second position, with both arms moving in tandem.

   b. Do 8 repetitions for each set.

4. **Flow into carriage of the arms (port de bras).**

   a. Begin with your arms in first position, maintaining a graceful shape, as if hugging a beach ball; your hands should be level with your navel, as shown earlier in Figure 7-11.

   b. Lift both arms to a high fifth position, maintaining your port de bras shape, and framing your face.

   c. Open your arms to second position, keeping them parallel to the floor in a T shape, but with a soft, slightly rounded form.

   d. Lower your arms to a low fifth position, framing the torso, keeping your hands level with your mid-thigh.

   e. Change direction.

   f. Do 8 repetitions for each set.

TIP

Familiarizing yourself with these essential Barre arm positions will make this exercise a breeze.

5. **Flow into the leg sequence (tendu).**

   a. Open your right leg to a second position plié and open your arms to second position.

   b. Close your left leg to a first position plié and bring your arms to first position.

   c. Open your right leg again to a second position plié and open your arms to second position.

   d. Lengthen both legs, keeping your weight on the right leg, and move your left leg to tendu, while bringing your arms to a high fifth position (Figure 7-12).

   e. Repeat in the other direction.

   f. Do 8 repetitions for each set.

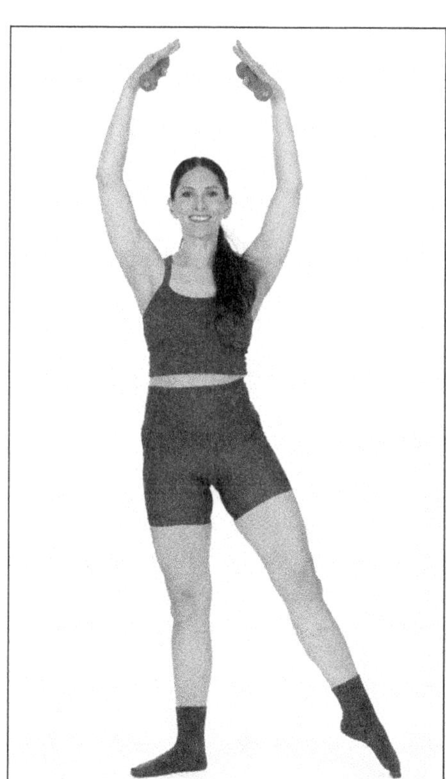

FIGURE 7-12:
Flow into the leg sequence (tendu).

Option 1: Passé

Repeat the leg sequence (tendu) in stage 5, lifting your left leg to passé at Step d. Do 8 repetitions in each set.

Option 2: Back attitude

Repeat the leg sequence (tendu) in stage 5, lifting your left leg to back attitude at step d, and placing your arms in first position. Do 8 repetitions for each set. Finish by pivoting your feet to parallel or open in second position.

Do's and don'ts

- » Do keep your abs activated, in and up.
- » Do maintain control through shoulder stabilization.
- » Do maintain control throughout.

Variations

- » Modify by skipping the weights.
- » Progress by adding a battement for the leg sequence (tendu).

Swimming and Temperature

This exercise focuses on the deltoids to strengthen the front and middle shoulders. You'll be doing a series of arm rotations, just like swimming, and "checking your temperature" by bringing the back of your hand to your forehead, hence the name. You'll need a set of light weights (tucked into the crook of your thumb joint with your fingers extended and relaxed), and you'll flow through eight movements. Do 8 to 16 repetitions for each set (up to 2 sets).

Getting set

Stand in the center of the floor with your arms out to the sides of your body in a T shape, parallel to the floor, palms facing forward.

The movement

The movement involves eight stages:

1. **Start with the single-arm swimming series.**

 a. Rotate your right shoulder internally until your right palm faces back. Think: "lift, roll, press," as shown in Figure 7-13.

 b. Rotate your right shoulder back to the start position, your right palm now facing forward again. Think: "lift, roll, lengthen."

 c. Repeat on the left side.

 d. Then, alternate right to left.

 e. Do 8 to 16 repetitions (up to 2 sets).

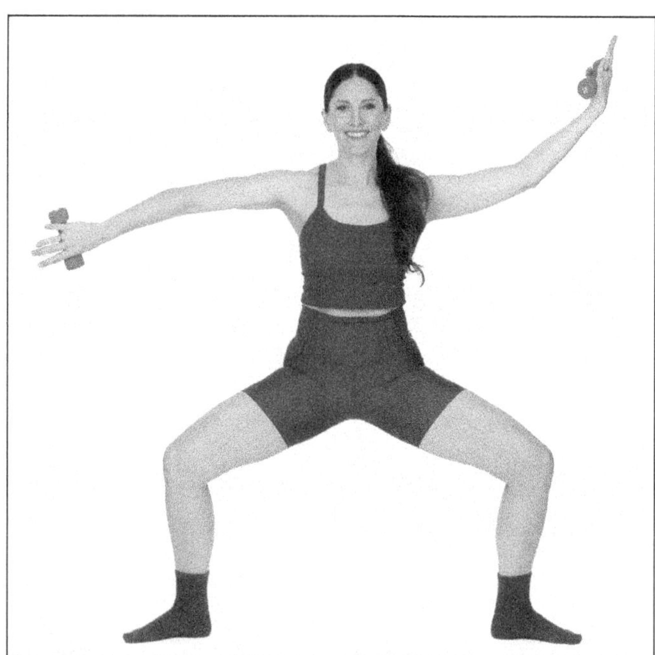

2. **Flow into the double-arm swimming series.**

 a. Repeat the series in stage 1 with your arms moving together in opposition.

 b. Do 8 to 16 repetitions (up to 2 sets).

3. **Flow into the single-arm temperature series.**

   a. Start with your arms in second position.

   b. Flow your right arm to first position.

   c. Lift and rotate your right arm so the back of your right hand nears your forehead (as if taking your temperature).

   d. Replace your right arm to first position, and then move it back to second position.

   e. Repeat on the left side.

   f. Do 8 to 16 repetitions (up to 2 sets).

4. **Flow into the double-arm temperature series.**

   a. Repeat the series in stage 3, but with arms both moving together.

   b. Do 8 to 16 repetitions (up to 2 sets).

5. **Flow into the dance series (lifts).**

   a. Lift your right arm to a high V, flexing from and leading with the wrist.

   b. Then, lower your arm to your side, extending the wrist.

   c. Repeat with your left arm, and then move both arms together.

   d. Do 8 to 16 repetitions (up to 2 sets).

6. **Flow into arm circles.**

   a. Keeping your wrists flexed and your arms out to the side and parallel with the floor, circle your arms in both directions.

   b. Repeat with your wrists extended.

   c. Do 8 to 16 repetitions (up to 2 sets).

7. **Flex and extend (aka the pom-pom push).**

   a. Bend your arms at the elbows, extending the wrists.

   b. Push your arms away, flexing the wrists, and repeat.

   c. Do 8 to 16 repetitions (up to 2 sets).

8. **Flow into diagonal arms.**

   a. Lift your right arm up to a high V, flexing from and leading with the wrist, while at the same time, lower your left arm to a low V, extending at the wrist.

   b. Slowly and mindfully alternate the move.

   c. Do 8 to 16 repetitions (up to 2 sets).

Finish by extending your arms even further.

Do's and don'ts

» Do keep your hips and shoulders square.

» Do maintain soft knees and elbows.

» Do keep your nonworking arm strong and lifted.

Variations

» Modify by omitting your weights and/or reducing your range of motion.

» Progress by using heavier weights.

V-Press

This classic press exercise focuses on your medial deltoids and lower trapezius muscles to strengthen the front and middle shoulders. And I added in some lunges for a compound movement focused on your thighs and glutes. You'll need a set of light weights (tucked into the crook of your thumb joint with your fingers extended and relaxed). Do 8 to 16 repetitions for each set.

Getting set

Stand in the center of the floor with your legs together, arms out to your sides and parallel to the floor, palms facing forward, with a slight bend in your knees and your abs activated.

The movement

The movement involves five stages:

1. **Start with a half V.**

   a. Lift both arms to a high V with your fingers extended.

   b. Return your arms to the start position.

    c. Lower your arms to a low V.

    d. Return your arms to the start position.

    e. Do 8 to 16 repetitions.

2. Flow into a full V.

    a. Lift your arms to a high V with your fingers extended.

    b. Lower your arms to a low V, and repeat.

    c. Do 8 to 16 repetitions.

3. Flow into a foundation rotation.

    a. Start with your arms in a high V with your palms facing inward and fingers extended.

    b. Rotate your torso to the right as your arms reach wide at your sides with your palms facing downward.

    c. Rotate back to the starting position and repeat on the other side.

    d. Do 8 to 16 repetitions.

4. Flow into a double rotation.

    a. Repeat the series in stage 3, but rotate your palms to face backward.

    b. Return to the start position.

    c. Repeat on the other side.

    d. Do 8 to 16 repetitions.

5. Flow into rotational wings.

    a. Start with your arms in a high V with your palms facing inward.

    b. Turn your body to the right and lunge forward with your right leg as your arms reach wide at your sides with your palms facing backward.

    c. Return to the start position.

    d. Repeat on the other side.

    e. Do 8 to 16 repetitions.

Finish with your arms by your sides.

Do's and don'ts

>> Do keep your hips square as your torso rotates.

>> Do maintain soft knees and elbows.

>> Do maintain shoulder stability when lifting your arms, and keep your shoulders down and relaxed.

Variations

>> Modify by omitting weights or reducing your range of motion.

>> Progress with heavier weights.

Rowing and Puppet

This exercise will have you moving your upper body in a rowing motion and your arms in a movement that'll make you feel like a puppet on a string. The muscle focus here is on posterior deltoids and rhomboids to develop shoulder and scapula stability. You'll need a set of light weights (tucked into the crook of your thumb joint with your fingers extended and relaxed). Do 8 to 16 repetitions for each set.

Getting set

Stand in the center of the floor. Begin with your arms lifted in front of your body, parallel to the floor like train tracks, with your palms facing down.

The movement

The movement involves two stages:

1. **Start with rowing.**

   a. Draw your arms back, parallel to the floor, opening your elbows to the sides of the room, as if you're pulling a set of oars.

   b. Return your arms to the start position and repeat.

c. Do 8 to 16 repetitions for each set.

Add a pulse back: With your elbows open to the sides of the room, carefully pulse your arms back, activating your posterior deltoids (be careful not to jam your shoulder blades together). Do 8 to 16 repetitions for each set.

2. **Flow into the puppet.**

   a. Start with your elbows open to the sides of the room, arms parallel to the floor (Figure 7-14).

   b. Rotate your arms to goalpost position — as if your hands are on strings — with your palms facing forward.

   c. Return your arms to the start position and repeat.

   d. Do 8 to 16 repetitions for each set.

Finish by stepping one leg back to lunge for hinge swing fly series.

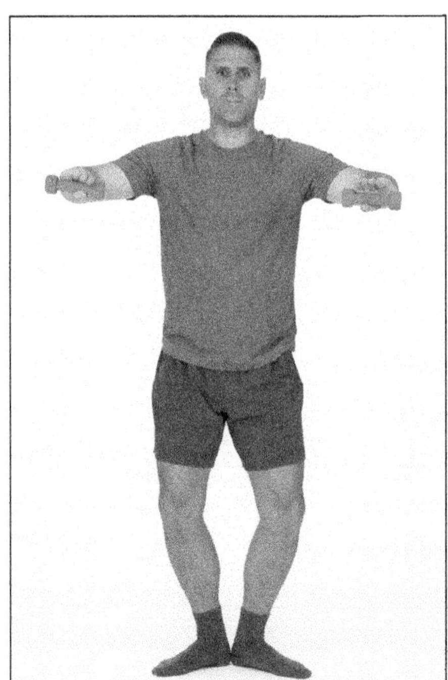

FIGURE 7-14: Start with your elbows open, arms parallel to the floor.

Do's and don'ts

» Do create your own resistance in each movement.

» Do maintain neutral shoulders.

» Do engage your core muscles.

Variations

» Modify by omitting your weights, and/or practice each segment separately for a more confident motion.

» Progress by concentrating on the flow from one set to the next without resting between sets.

» Add a plié/relevé with arm actions. (Why not?)

Hinge Swing Fly Series

The hinge swing fly series focuses on testing and developing your coordination while working your shoulders, triceps, and abdominals. You'll need a set of light weights (tucked into the crook of your thumb joint with your fingers extended and relaxed), and you'll be doing 8 to 16 repetitions for each set.

Getting set

Stand in the center of the floor with your feet together. Bend your knees and hinge at the crease of your thighs, leaning forward to form a diagonal line from the top of your head to your seat.

The movement

The movement involves two stages:

1. **Start with a pulse up.**

   a. Reach your right arm forward with your palm facing down, and then extend your left arm backward with your palm facing up.

   b. Pulse your arms upward three times.

c. Open your arms to second position.

d. Alternate sides and repeat.

e. Do 8 to 16 repetitions for each set.

2. **Finish with a pulse in.**

a. Reach your right arm forward with your palm facing down, and then extend your left arm backward with your palm facing up.

b. Pulse your arms inward three times toward the midline.

c. Alternate sides and repeat.

d. Do 8 to 16 repetitions for each set.

Your palms can be facing inward in both actions.

Finish with one arm back and extend the same leg, ready for curtsy triceps.

Do's and don'ts

» Do allow your shoulders to hang down with your neck long.

» Do concentrate on maintaining a neutral spine.

» Do keep your hips and shoulders square.

Variations

» Modify by decreasing your range of motion.

» Progress by increasing repetitions and/or using heavier weights.

Curtsy Triceps

Although this exercise targets the triceps, it also develops torso and scapula stabilization while focusing on lower-body stabilization with a curtsy-like lunge. You'll need a set of light weights (tucked into the crook of your thumb joint with your fingers extended and relaxed), and you'll be doing 8 to 16 repetitions for each set.

Getting set

Stand in the center of the floor with your arms and legs in a second position plié. Hinge from the crease of your thighs, reach your sit bones to the back wall, and lean forward. Flow your arms up to a high fifth position, framing the face, as shown in Figure 7-15.

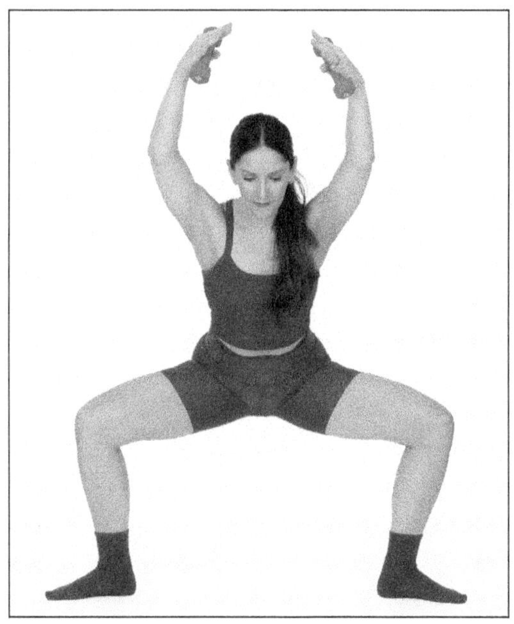

Your *sit bones* are the two bony points at the base of your pelvis that you feel when sitting upright on a firm surface. In Barre, grounding through your sit bones helps you stay stable, aligned, and supported, especially during seated or floor exercises. Good to have them in mind.

TECHNICAL STUFF

The movement

The movement involves three stages:

1. **Start with curtsy triceps.**

   a. Step your right leg back to a curtsy lunge as both arms hug to a low fifth position behind your torso, framing the back.

   b. Open to a second position plié as your arms return to a high fifth position.

c. Then, step your left leg back to a curtsy lunge as both arms hug to a low fifth position behind your torso, framing your back.

d. Open to second position plié as your arms return to a high fifth position.

e. Repeat.

f. Do 8 to 16 repetitions for each position (up to 2 sets).

This is a moving cardio sequence that can be used between two sets of triceps lunges in the curtsy position.

2. **Flow into arms in and up.**

   a. In a curtsy lunge, press your arms inward toward each other, then pulse your arms up for the next set.

   b. Do 8 to 16 repetitions for each position (up to 2 sets).

3. **Bend and extend.**

   a. In a curtsy lunge, flex your elbows, keeping your humerus still.

   b. Extend your elbows back to the start position and repeat.

   c. Do 8 to 16 repetitions for each position (up to 2 sets).

Finish open to second position, take a deep breath in and out, and bring your legs together, ready for Triceps Lunges.

Do's and don'ts

» Do keep equal weight distribution on your feet.

» Do keep your arms up in second position and down in curtsy.

» Do keep your hips and shoulders square.

Variations

» Modify by starting slow before increasing tempo.

» Progress by adding pulses in curtsy position during arm variations and/ or adding plié tendu extension of the back leg in stage C.

Triceps Lunges

Although this lunge exercise series targets the triceps, it also develops torso and scapular stabilization while focusing on lower-body stabilization and strengthening the triceps. You'll need a set of light weights (tucked into the crook of your thumb joint with your fingers extended and relaxed), and you'll be doing 8 to 16 repetitions for each set. If you like, you can leave out one of the movements in stages 2, 3, or 4, or try all three if you're feeling powerful.

Getting set

Stand in the center of the floor in a parallel stance, lift your right leg to passé and lift your right leg behind as the left leg bends, hinging from the crease of the thigh, leaning forward. Create a long diagonal line from the top of your head to your toes, as shown in Figure 7-16. Either use the same arm as the extended leg with the other arm resting on your thigh for stability, or use both arms, lengthen to the sides of your pelvis.

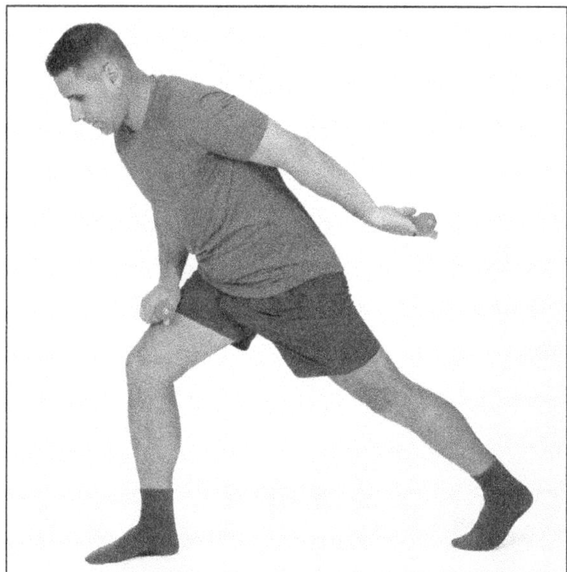

FIGURE 7-16: Step back into a triceps lunge.

The movement

The movement involves five stages:

1. **Start with a press-up.**

   a. Lift your working arm(s) above the level of your pelvis.

   b. Return to the start position and repeat.

   c. Increase the tempo to pulses and repeat.

   d. Do 8 to 16 repetitions for each position (up to 2 sets).

2. **Flow into arm circles.**

   a. Maintaining your hinged-forward position, circle the working arm(s) with emphasis on the "in" and "up."

   b. Reverse the direction of the circles.

   c. Do 8 to 16 repetitions for each position (up to 2 sets).

Keep the circles small, around 10 inches in circumference.

TIP

3. **Flow into a side to back.**

   a. Maintaining your hinged-forward position, and with your palm(s) facing in, open your working arm(s) to the side (in line with your pelvis).

   b. Then, draw back to the start position and repeat.

      Optional add-on: Add a press-up once your arm(s) return(s) to the start position. Think: "open, close, lift, lower."

   c. Do 8 to 16 repetitions for each position (up to 2 sets).

4. **Flow into flex and extend.**

   a. Maintaining your hinged-forward position, flex and extend your working arm(s), keeping the humerus (upper arm) lifted. (**Note:** The flex is small; concentrate on extending the arms to really engage the triceps.)

   b. Choose two to three exercises from stages 2 to 4, and alternate sides if performing the single arm option.

   c. Do 8 to 16 repetitions for each position (up to 2 sets).

5. **Flow into a black swan.**

   a. Reach both arms to a low V with your palms facing in, just above the level of your pelvis.

b. Sweep your arms out to second position, undulating the arms like swan wings, and repeat.

c. Do 8 to 16 repetitions for each position (up to 2 sets).

Finish by lifting up one more inch and then lowering, bringing your legs together.

Do's and don'ts

» Do square off your hips and shoulders.

» Do keep your shoulders and hips parallel.

» Do work on equal weight distribution on the supporting foot, so keep an eye on your foot and knee alignment.

Variations

» Modify by performing each series slowly before increasing the tempo.

» Progress with a deeper lunge, and/or lift the back foot off the floor.

Chapter **8**

Barre Work Basics: The Classic Positions

The classic moves covered in this chapter are the heart of your Barre workout. They are designed to target the lower-body muscle groups, beginning with the front of the thigh (quadriceps) and ending with the back of the thigh (hamstrings and glutes). The exercises in this chapter help you transition seamlessly from sculpt to cardio, then back to sculpt and stretch. Master each exercise, and you can achieve a well-choreographed, nonstop series that truly flows.

Exercises in This Chapter

The exercises in this chapter include the following:

» First-Position Pliés

» Second-Position Pliés

» Fourth Position

» Second-Position Cardio

» Parallel Pliés

>> Hip Circles

>> Passé Press Series

>> Back to Barre Battements

>> Back Attitude

>> Ballet Lunges

>> Hamstring Series

>> Side Lifts

>> Resistance Band Series

>> Fold-Over Series

For each exercise, I first help you prepare, and then I provide detailed steps for each one, followed by do's and don'ts to keep in mind as you practice. Finally, each section ends with ideas for variation.

To complete the exercises in this chapter, you need a ball, a light hand weight, and a resistance band.

TIP

First-Position Pliés

This exercise focuses on your quadriceps to strengthen your buttocks, thighs, calves, ankles, and feet. It helps improve balance, too.

Getting set

Stand tall with one hand on your barre for support and your free arm in a port de bras position — a soft, rounded, and graceful shape with the elbow lifted and wrist and fingers gently extended — and your feet together (see Figure 8-1). Rock gently onto your heels and open your feet to first position or into a "natural turnout," with your toes approximately 6 to 10 inches apart, heels together, and knees soft. Get ready to plié and extend, bend and extend, and lower and lift.

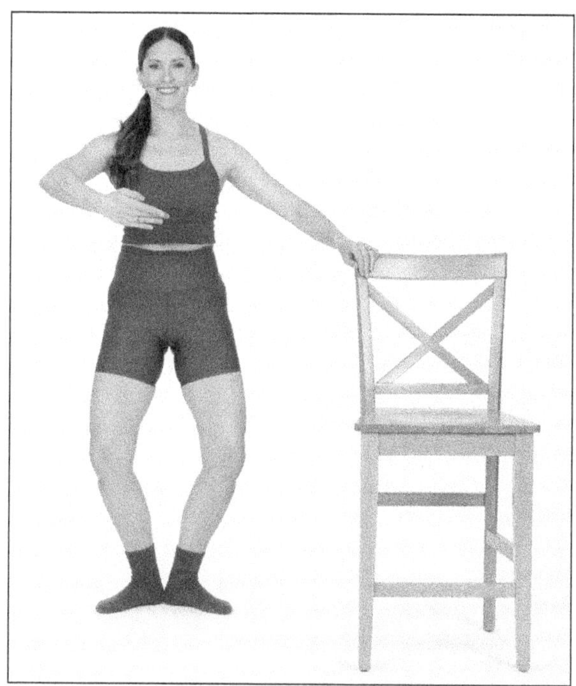

The movement

This movement involves four stages:

1. Begin with pliés.

a. Gently bend both knees and lower your body down, keeping both heels firmly connected to the floor and each other.

b. Engage your inner thighs to extend your legs, and gently rise to your starting position, keeping your knees slightly bent.

c. Do 8 to 16 repetitions.

2. Switch to narrow pliés.

a. Place your feet in a narrow first position with your toes approximately 3 inches apart, heels together, and knees soft.

b. Bend your knees into a half-plié and lift heels high, raising onto the balls of your feet and keeping your heels firmly connected.

c. Lower into a deeper bend — your challenge zone — and begin to lower and lift.

d. Maintain your foot position (on the balls of your feet, heels lifted and connected) as you repeat for 8 to 16 pliés.

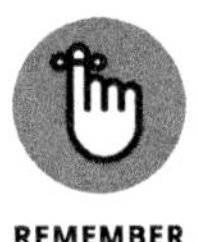

Your *challenge zone* is the point where you're pushing yourself without risk of injury.

3. **Flow into pliés on relevé.**

   a. Hold your plié and keep your body still.

   b. Raise both heels high, allowing them to separate as you lift the heels away from the floor (Figure 8-2).

   c. With control, lower your body down and back up as you stay in your challenge zone.

   d. Repeat for 8 to 16 repetitions (up to 2 sets).

4. **End with heel lifts.**

   a. Hold the plié position and keep your body still.

   b. Lift both heels up to a high relevé (where they will naturally separate).

   c. Articulate the heels down so your heels reconnect and touch the floor.

   d. Continue to lift and lower your heels on and off the floor, staying in your challenge zone.

   e. Repeat for 8 to 16 repetitions (up to 2 sets).

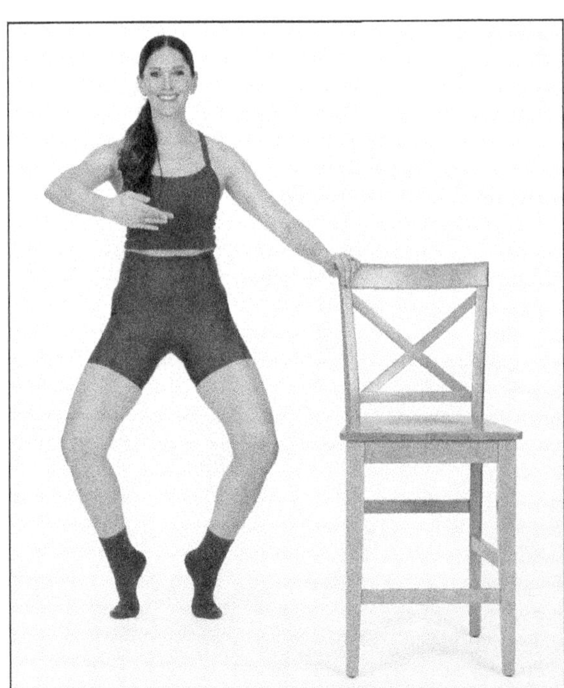

FIGURE 8-2: Raise both heels high, allowing them to separate naturally.

Do's and don'ts

>> Do keep your shoulders over your hips and your hips over your heels.

>> Do press through the heels on plié and engage your abdominal muscles.

>> Do maintain soft elbows.

>> Don't grip the barre; gently rest your hand on the barre for support.

>> Don't force turnout; keep your knees soft and over the second and third toes.

Variations

>> Modify by decreasing the number of repetitions, the number of sets, and the range of motion. Skip stage 3 (pliés on relevé), if needed.

>> Progress by increasing your range of motion and the number of repetitions and/or sets.

Second-Position Pliés

This exercise is a wide plié with three stages that focus on your quadriceps and calves to lengthen and strengthen your inner and outer thighs and encourage hip mobility. Use one arm or both for stability.

Getting set

Stand sideways at the barre. Use one hand for support and hold your free arm in a port de bras position. (For more support, face the barre and use both hands for extra stability.) Stand tall with your feet slightly wider than shoulder distance. Rock gently onto your heels and open your feet to second position with a natural turnout. Get ready to plié and extend, lower and lift.

The movement

This movement involves three stages:

1. **Start with pliés.**

   a. Bend your knees into a deep second position plié (Figure 8-3), and hold in your challenge zone for 8 counts.

   b. Press through your heels and engage your abdominal muscles to extend your legs back up, squeezing your seat, inner thighs, and hamstrings.

   c. Repeat two sets of 8 repetitions.

2. **Flow into pliés on relevé.**

   a. Plié into a deep second position, hold in your challenge zone, and keep your body stable.

   b. Lift your right heel and pulse your body up and down with a small movement as you keep your heel up, as shown in Figure 8-3. Do 8 to 16 repetitions.

   c. Repeat with your left heel.

   d. Do 8 to 16 repetitions on both sides.

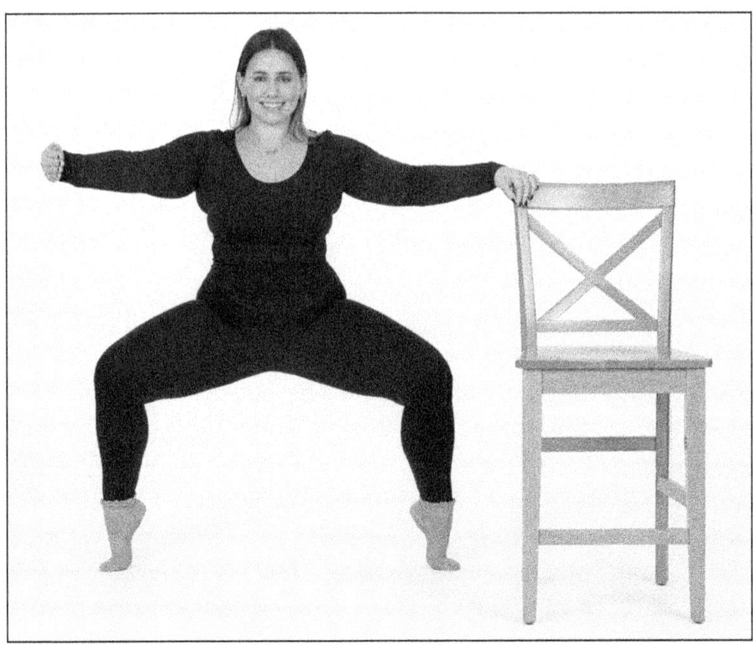

FIGURE 8-3:
A Second Position plié in relevé.

3. **Finish with heel lifts.**

    a. Plié into a deep second position, hold in your challenge zone, and keep your body stable.

    b. Switch between lifting your left heel and your right heel.

    c. Repeat two sets of 8 repetitions.

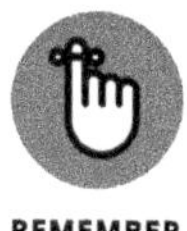

Only lift one heel at a time and keep your body still and controlled.

  Finish by standing tall, ready for fourth position.

Do's and don'ts

>> Do keep your hips and shoulders square and your abdominals in.

>> Do align your knees over your first two toes.

>> Don't bounce through the pliés; create a smooth flow instead.

>> Don't force the knees open; allow them to turn out naturally from the hips.

Variations

>> Modify by keeping your heels down and decreasing the range of motion or number of repetitions.

>> Progress by increasing the range of motion or the number of repetitions.

>> To further advance, add pliés as you lift your heels.

Fourth Position

This exercise challenges your core stability by focusing on your trunk and gluteus muscles to strengthen the lower body. Do 8 to 16 repetitions and up to 2 sets. Repeat the series on the other side.

Getting set

Stand sideways at the barre, using one hand for support and holding your free arm in a port de bras position. Stand tall. Rock gently onto your heels and open your feet to first position or "natural turnout." Then, step your outside leg back to fourth position, as shown in Figure 8-4. Get ready to bend and extend.

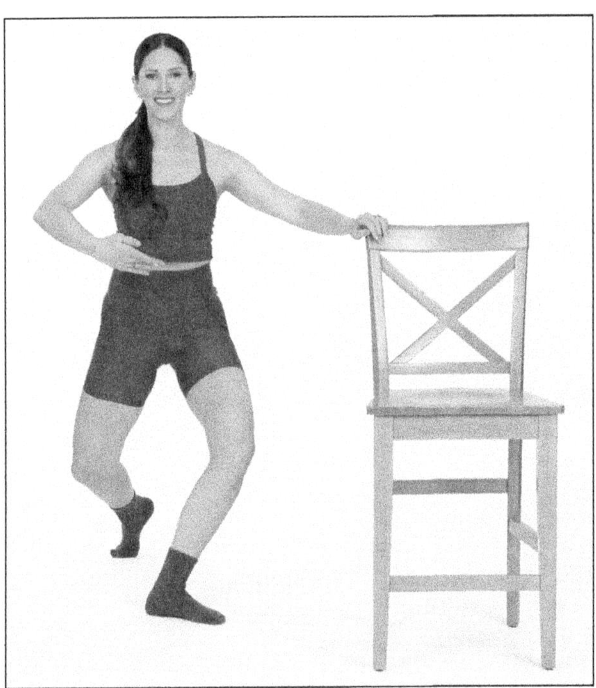

The movement

This movement involves three stages:

1. **Start with a plié.**

   a. Bend your knees to potential, keeping your front heel connected to the floor.

   b. Extend your legs and rise up while engaging your inner thighs and seat muscles.

   c. Do 8 to 16 repetitions.

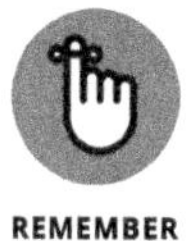

2. Bending your knees to potential means lowering only as far as you can while keeping good alignment. Your heels stay grounded, your knees track over your toes, and your spine stays upright. Go as deep as feels strong and controlled, never forced.

3. **Flow into front heel lifts.**

   a. Holding your plié, lift your front heel up and then lower it back down to the floor.

   b. Do 8 to 16 repetitions.

4. **Finish with a plié on relevé.**

   a. Bend both knees to your lowest plié, lift both heels, and lower and lift the position (Figure 8-5).

   b. Do 8 to 16 repetitions (up to 2 sets).

Finish with a hold in your lowest plié and repeat on the other side.

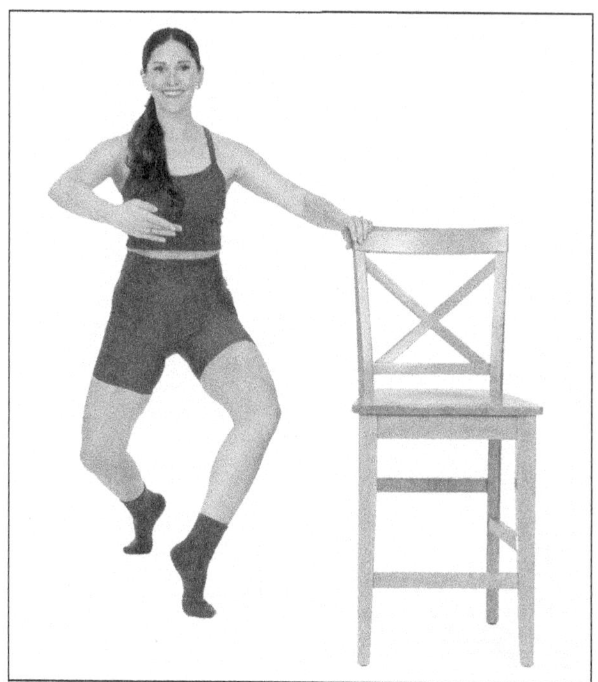

FIGURE 8-5:
Bend both knees, lift both heels; lower and lift.

Do's and don'ts

>> Do keep your hips and shoulders square.

>> Do focus on single-leg strength.

>> Do flow from one movement into the next.

>> Do keep your supporting leg in relevé throughout the series.

Variations

>> Modify by omitting the relevés.

>> Progress by increasing your range of motion or complete with both heels in relevé.

Second-Position Cardio

Through cardio movement, this exercise focuses on the quadriceps to increase coordination and body awareness while strengthening your inner and outer thighs and encouraging hip mobility. Get ready to raise your heart rate, plié, and sweep!

Getting set

Stand sideways at the barre. Use one hand for support and hold your free arm in a port de bras position and stand tall. Rock gently onto your heels and open your feet to second position.

The movement

This movement involves three stages:

1. **Start with second position to straight leg.**

   a. Plié in second position, as shown in Figure 8-6.

   b. Sweep your outside arm and leg toward your body, crossing the midline as you gently straighten your supporting leg.

   c. Move your arm and leg back out to the front of your body into first position.

   d. Do two sets of 8 repetitions.

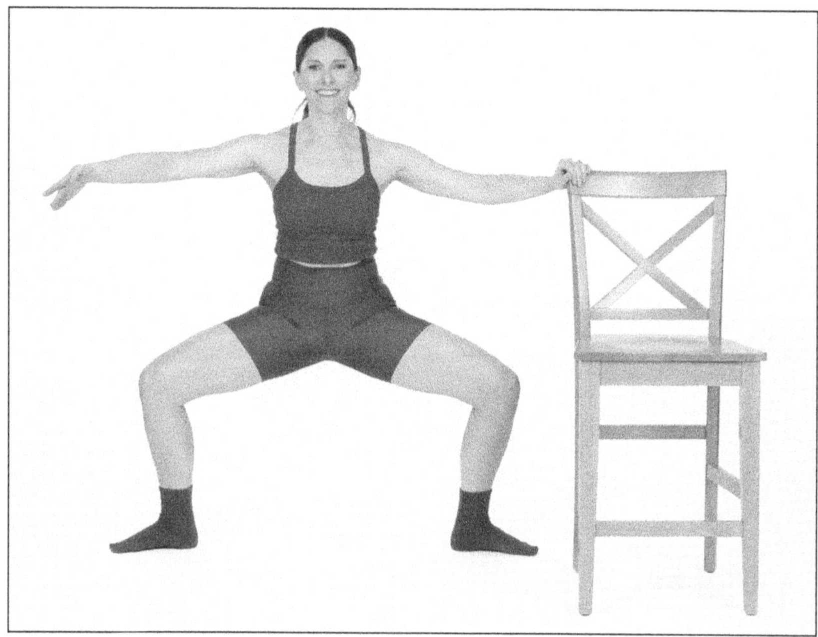

2. **Flow into second position to attitude.**

   a. Plié in second position.

   b. Sweep your arm high overhead and your leg into a front attitude position (Figure 8-7) as you gently straighten your supporting leg.

   c. Do two sets of 8 repetitions.

3. **Finally, flow into second position to battement.**

   a. Plié in second position.

   b. Keep your arm in second position and bring your working leg to a side battement as your supporting leg straightens.

   c. Do two sets of 8 repetitions.

Finish by turning to your other side to repeat.

Do's and don'ts

» Do disassociate your upper body from your lower body. This will help to maintain correct alignment for each exercise.

» Do keep your hips and shoulders square.

» Do follow natural turnout as you kick during stage 3.

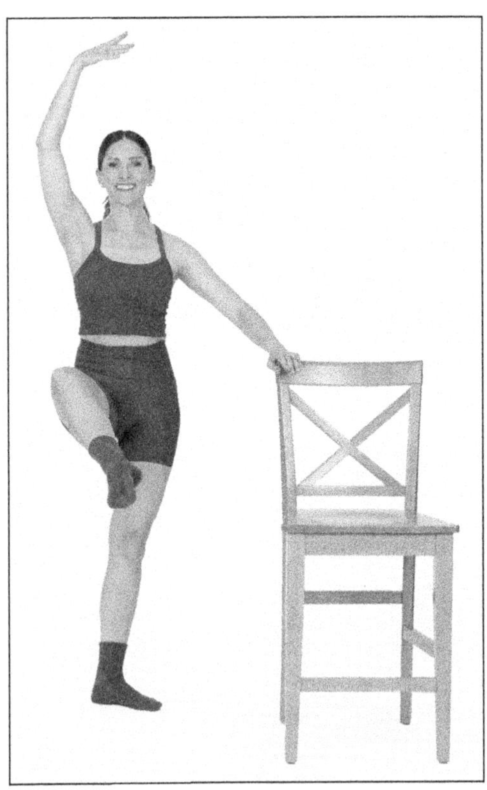

Variations

>> Modify by starting with only one set, and/or decreasing your range of motion.

>> Progress by adding relevé on your inside heel as you straighten your leg and/or increase your range of motion.

Parallel Pliés

This exercise focuses on the quadriceps to align and stabilize the hips, strengthen the lower body, and improve pelvic control and stabilization. Grab your ball and get ready to bend and extend.

Getting set

Stand at the barre facing forward or sideways with your feet parallel and legs together. Relevé so that your heels lift off the floor, keeping your heels high and connected. Plié down to a position where your knees are over your toes and your hips are just over your heels, as shown in Figure 8-8. Use your inner thighs to maintain connection with your legs.

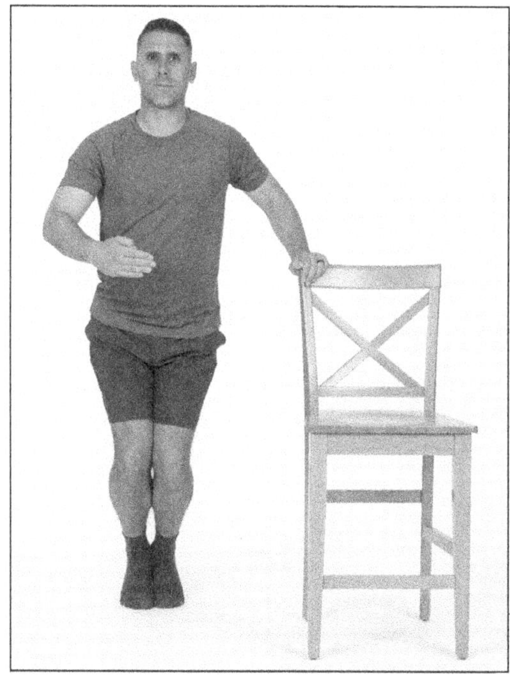

FIGURE 8-8: Lift your heels and plié down where your knees are over your toes.

The movement

This movement involves three stages:

1. **Start with a plié on relevé.**

   a. Hold this position with no movement for 8 counts to focus on your posture and placement.

   b. Then, plié down and up within a few inches, never rising above your challenge zone.

   c. Do 8 to 16 repetitions.

2. **Flow into a ball pulse.**

   a. Place a ball between your inner thighs.

   b. Relevé your heels up and plié down to your challenge zone.

   c. Holding this position, pulse the ball using your inner thighs (place the ball above the knees).

   d. Squeeze 8 slow pulses, then 16 at a slightly faster tempo.

   e. Lower your body down 1 inch and pulse the ball, then lift up 1 inch and pulse the ball.

   f. Continue for 8 repetitions.

   g. Hold in your challenge zone and repeat the ball pulse (8 slow pulses, 16 quick).

   h. Finish with a relevé up to starting position and lower your heels.

3. **Finish with hip isolation.**

   a. Relevé your heels and plié to your challenge zone, as shown in Figure 8-9.

   b. Draw your tailbone under, bringing your pubic bone to your navel (posterior tilt), and engage your lower abdominals.

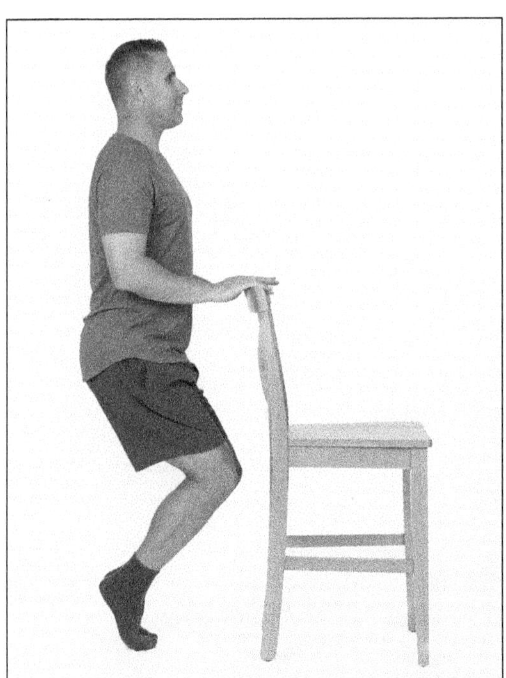

FIGURE 8-9: Relevé your heels and plié to your challenge zone.

c. Repeat, using both slow and quicker tempos.

d. Reach the right side of your pelvis toward the barre, as if trying to touch the barre.

e. Return to starting position and repeat on the left side.

f. Alternate, utilize both slow and quicker tempos.

g. Do 8 to 16 repetitions (up to 2 sets).

Do's and don'ts

» Do think about your posture and your body alignment — your shoulders over your hips, and your hips over your heels.

» Do keep your heels lifted to support and strengthen the muscles surrounding the knees.

» Do hold your abdominals in to support your lower back.

» Do keep your knees, inner thighs, and heels connected.

» Don't bend at the waist; maintain a tall spine.

Variations

» Modify by making your pliés very small, or use no movement at all; just hold the position.

» Progress by increasing your range of motion and/or the number of repetitions.

» Progress further by lifting both hands off the barre to a high fifth position and maintaining your balance.

Hip Circles

This exercise focuses on your quadriceps to align and stabilize your hips and strengthen your quads while focusing on pelvic control and stabilization. Do 8 repetitions and up to 2 sets.

Getting set

Stand at the barre facing forward or sideways. With your feet together in parallel, relevé, keeping your heels high, and plié down to a position where your knees are over your toes and your hips are over your heels.

The movement

This movement involves three stages:

1. **Start with isolation.**

   a. Relevé, lifting both heels, and plié down to your challenge zone.

   b. Draw your tailbone under, bringing your pubic bone to your navel as you engage seat muscles and contract your abdominals.

   c. Repeat 8 tucks slowly and 16 tucks at tempo.

   d. Hold the position and begin to tuck your pubic bone under (posterior tilt), moving your hips from right to left, reaching to "touch" the right and left hip bone toward the barre.

   e. Do 8 repetitions.

2. **Flow into circles.**

   a. Hold the position in your challenge zone and begin to circle your hips to the right for 8 repetitions (Figure 8-10).

   b. Repeat with circles to the left for 8 repetitions.

   c. Reduce to 4 repetitions in each direction.

   d. Reduce to 2 repetitions in each direction.

3. **Finish with a corkscrew.**

   a. Circle your hips two times to the right as you deepen your plié.

   b. Reverse the circles to swivel back up to starting position.

   c. Do 2 repetitions in each direction.

Finish with a relevé up and lower down.

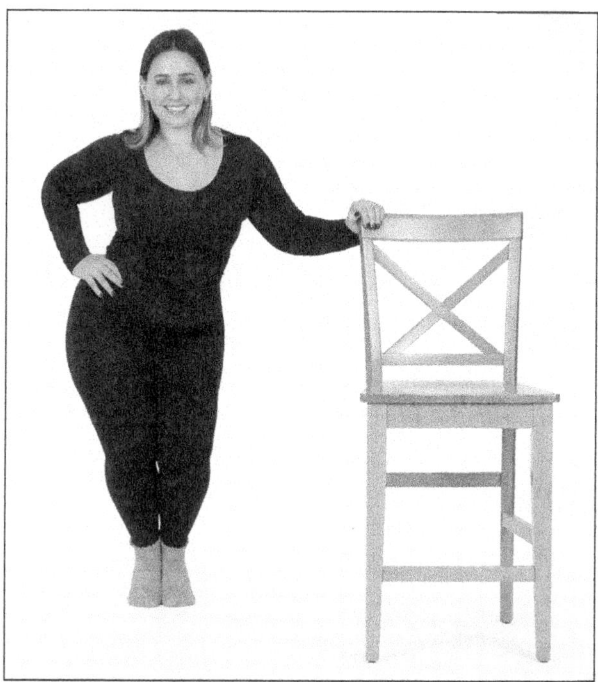

Do's and don'ts

>> Do keep your shoulders stacked over your hips.

>> Do keep your heels up to support and strengthen the muscles surrounding your knees.

>> Do maintain a tall spine; do not bend at the waist.

>> Do pull in your abdominals to support your lower back.

Variations

>> Modify by making your pliés small, or do no movement at all; just hold the position.

>> Just starting out? Start with 8 repetitions and slowly advance to the entire series.

>> Progress by increasing your range of motion and/or the number of repetitions.

Passé Press Series

This exercise focuses on the quadriceps, hamstrings, and adductors (outer thighs) to increase coordination and body awareness while strengthening the inner and outer thighs and encouraging hip mobility. Do 8 repetitions for each set, up to 2 sets. Get ready to plié and passé, press and lift.

Getting set

Standing sideways to the barre, open your arms. Rock gently onto your heels and open your feet to second position.

The movement

1. **Start with second position to passé.**

   a. Plié deep in second position.

   b. Press your right foot off the floor to your left knee (a passé), balancing on your left leg.

   c. Step to deep second position and repeat.

   d. Do 8 to 16 repetitions.

2. **Finish with pirouette prep.**

   a. Turned out, plié your inside leg as you extend your outside arm and leg in opposition (Figure 8-11).

   b. Straighten your supporting leg as you draw your working leg into a side passé and your arm into fifth position (Figure 8-12).

   c. Repeat 8 slowly and then 8 repetitions at tempo.

Finish by holding your balance or crossing your ankle to the other side and holding your balance.

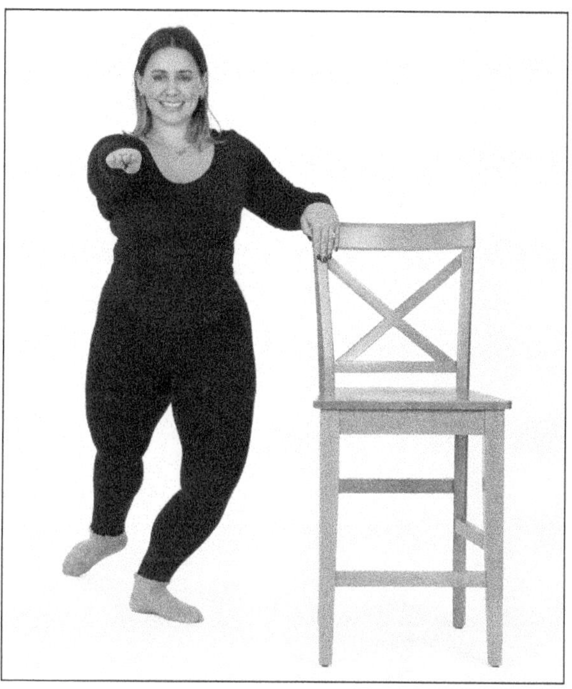

Do's and don'ts

>> Do maintain a neutral spine, especially as you extend your arm and leg.

>> Do engage your seat muscles as you extend your leg behind your body and on relevé leg.

>> Do maintain a strong focus on your arm placement — full extension in front of your shoulder.

>> Do remember to resist as you draw your arm into first position.

Variations

>> Modify by omitting the relevé, taking the pirouette prep into parallel, and/or decreasing your range of motion.

>> Progress by adding relevé and/or increasing your range of motion.

>> To advance, add a relevé with your supporting leg as you passé. Your hands can be lifted to high fifth on passé to further challenge your balance.

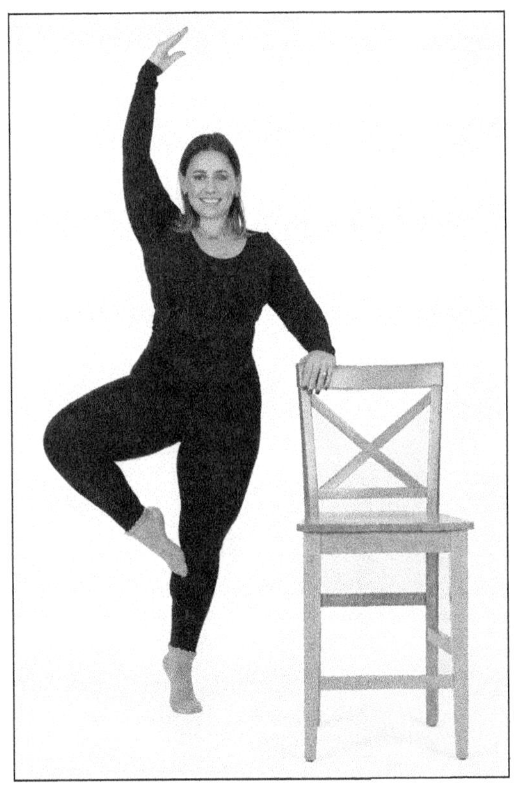

Back to Barre Battements

This exercise focuses on the quadriceps to improve your hip flexors and strengthen your quads while stabilizing your supporting seat muscles. Do 8 repetitions for each set, up to 2 sets. Get ready to kick and resist.

Getting set

Stand tall with your back to the barre, with your feet together in parallel stance or turned out in first position. Place your arms on the barre behind you with a wide overhand grip if possible.

The movement

This movement involves three stages:

1. **Start with battement.**

   a. Point one foot in front of your body (Figure 8-13).

   b. Lift your foot, inch by inch, to your fullest potential (Figure 8-14).

   c. Once your potential height is reached, lower your leg back down with control.

   d. Keep a nice flow, extending your leg up in the air and lowering it back down to the floor with control. Repeat on the other leg.

   e. Do 8 repetitions.

2. **Flow into passé.**

   a. Keep your leg up, bend your knee into passé, and extend it back out.

   b. Maintain upper-body control as you bend and extend your leg, engaging your abdominals to assist.

   c. Do 8 repetitions.

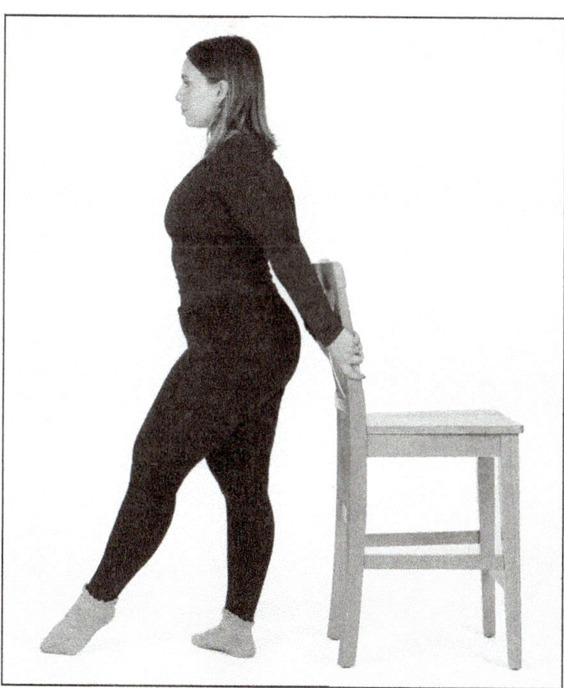

FIGURE 8-13: With your back to the barre, point your foot.

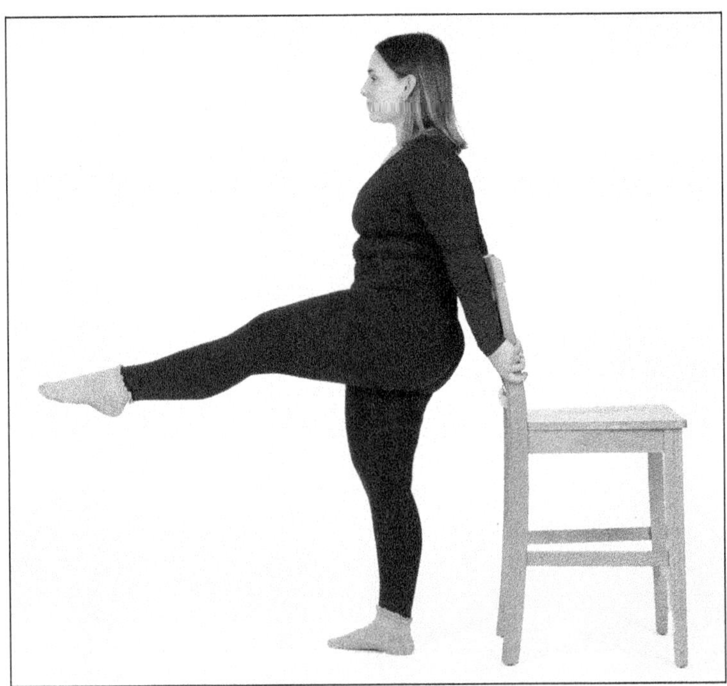

3. **Finish with attitude.**

   a. Keep your leg up and bend your knee into attitude and extend it back out. Turn away from the barre if you need more space.

   b. Maintain upper-body control as you bend and extend your leg, engaging your abdominals to assist.

   c. Do 8 repetitions.

Finish by either stretching your quads or performing an oppositional exercise at the barre. Then, pivot to face the barre.

Do's and don'ts

» Do keep your abdominals in and your shoulders down.

» Do stand tall on your supporting leg.

» Don't hunch forward.

» Don't lean back into the barre to lift your leg higher; work within your limits.

Variations

» Modify by keeping your range of motion small.

» Progress by extending your fingers, pressing the heels of your hands into the barre, and adding pulses on the last repetition. Keep your leg up in the air and pulse up 8 quick times. Alternate sides.

Back Attitude

This exercise focuses on the gluteus medius, hamstrings, and quads to align and stabilize the hips while strengthening your seat and toning your hamstrings and thighs. Do 8 repetitions slowly or 16 fast. Grab your hand weight and get ready to lift and lower.

Getting set

Face the barre, standing tall, feet in first position. Demi plié (with both heels on the floor), place your weight onto one foot, and extend your other leg into a back attitude, as shown in Figure 8-15.

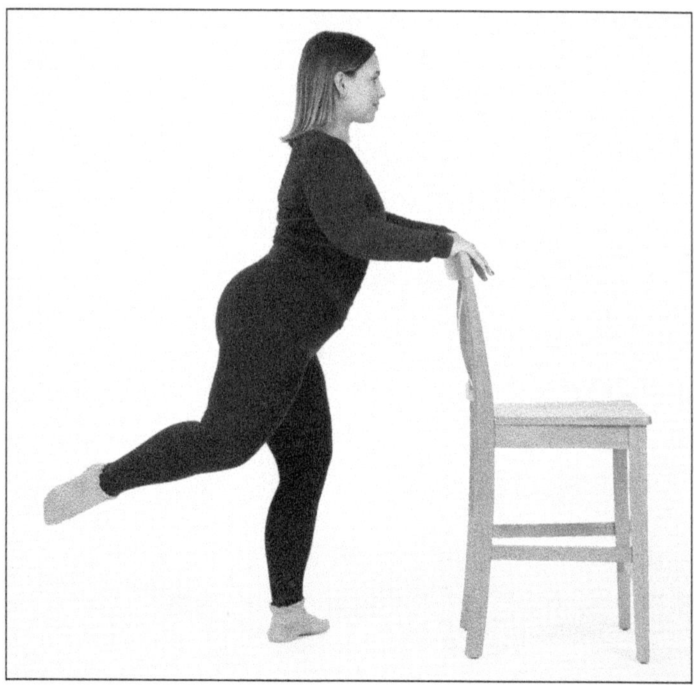

FIGURE 8-15: Facing the barre, place weight onto one foot and bend your working leg into a back attitude.

The movement

This movement involves five stages:

1. **Start with a knee lift.**

   a. With leg in back attitude, lift and lower your knee with control.

   b. Use your seat muscles, not your knees, to initiate movement.

   c. Do 8 slow repetitions or 16 fast.

2. **Then, flow into a press back.**

   a. Bend your working leg into back attitude and press your thigh back in small, controlled movements.

   b. Maintain a turned-out position.

   c. Do 8 slow repetitions or 16 fast.

3. **Flow into a combination.**

   a. Combine a knee lift with a press back (stages 1 and 2).

   b. Press back, and then gently lift your knee up, keeping your hips square.

   c. Do 8 slow repetitions or 16 fast.

4. **Flow into a midline pulse.**

   a. With your leg in a back attitude, pulse to cross the midline of the body.

   b. Use your inner thigh muscles, not your knees, to initiate movement.

   c. Do 8 slow repetitions or 16 fast.

5. **Finish with double attitude.**

   a. Deepen your plié on your supporting leg as your working leg bends to attitude.

   b. Extend both legs together.

   c. Do 8 to 16 repetitions.

Finish by lifting one more inch.

Do's and don'ts

» Do not lean into your supporting leg.

» Do maintain your weight over your heels, not toes. This will help to put the movement into your seat and not your knees.

>> Do keep your hips square, pressing slightly toward the barre.

>> Do keep the supporting leg bent as your hips press forward and your thigh presses back.

Variations

>> Modify by decreasing your range of motion.

>> Progress by adding relevé, increasing your range of motion and/or the number of repetitions.

Ballet Lunges

This exercise focuses on the gluteus medius, hamstrings, and quads to align and stabilize your hips while strengthening your seat and toning your hamstrings and thighs. Do 8 repetitions slowly or 16 fast. Get ready to slide and return.

Getting set

Stand tall, facing the barre with your feet parallel and together, and your hands holding the barre with an underhanded grip. Place the top of your right foot behind your body.

The movement

This movement involves three stages:

1. **Start with a lunge.**

   a. Slide your right foot behind your body (keeping your leg as straight as possible) as your left leg moves into a lunge.

   b. Return to standing without putting any weight on your right foot.

   c. Repeat this series, doing 8 to 16 repetitions.

2. **Flow into lower and lifts.**

   a. Hold the lunge position.

   b. Perform 8 small plié pulses and 8 heel taps.

3. **Finish with a standing leg pulse.**

   a. Hold the lunge position and transfer your weight forward to lean on a slight diagonal.

   b. Lift your leg to potential and pulse up for 16 repetitions.

Finish by drawing your legs together in relevé and lower down.

Do's and don'ts

>> Do make sure your back leg is straight; this is not a curtsy shape or traditional lunge.

>> Do be mindful to perfectly track the knee; the angle of the joint needs to be 90 degrees so that your *muscles* bring you out of the lunge, not your joints.

Variations

>> Modify by decreasing your range of motion.

>> Progress by increasing your range of motion and/or the number of repetitions.

>> Perform in relevé.

Hamstring Series

This exercise focuses on the hamstrings to strengthen your seat and tone the back of your legs. Do 8 repetitions slowly or 16 fast. Grab your ball and get ready to press and resist, back and in.

Getting set

Stand tall, or fold at the waist, and face the barre. Open your feet to hip distance and place a ball behind the knee of one leg. Soften the knee of your supporting leg, as shown in Figure 8-16.

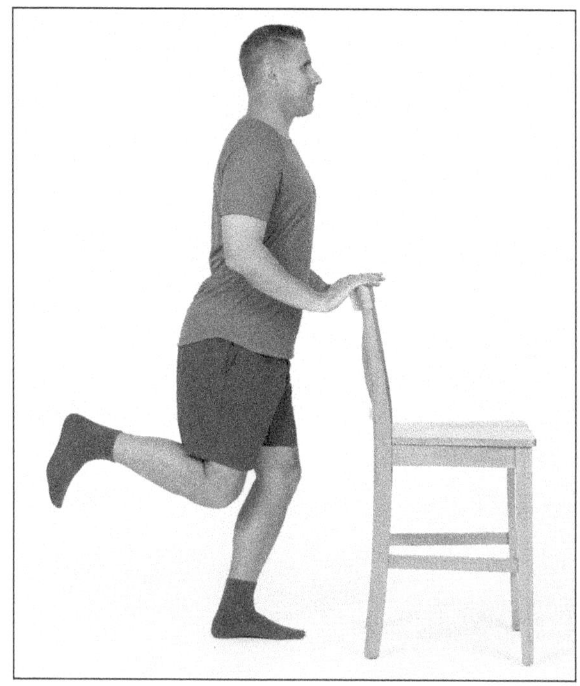

The movement

This movement involves three stages:

1. **Start with a press back.**

   a. Press your working leg back behind the other knee.

   b. Press your knee and ball back for 16 repetitions, maintaining a slight posterior pelvic tilt.

   c. Hold your leg back and pulse the ball 8 times slowly, then 16 times quickly.

2. **Flow into a side lift.**

   a. Open your working leg to the side while engaging the ball.

   b. Lower and lift your leg for 8 repetitions.

   c. Hold at the top or side position and pulse your leg up for 8 repetitions.

   d. Hold your leg to the side and pulse the ball 8 times slowly, then 16 quickly.

3. **Flow into circles.**

   a. Keeping your knee lifted to the side, begin to circle your leg.

   b. Circle 4 to 8 times in each direction

4. **Repeat the series on the other leg.**

Finish by standing tall to the side of the barre, ready for side lifts.

Do's and don'ts

>> Do maintain a slight bend in the supporting leg.

>> Don't hyperextend; be mindful.

>> Do press your hips forward as your thigh presses back.

>> Do make sure your hips are square to the barre; do not lift them.

>> Do keep your shoulders over your hips with a neutral spine.

Variations

>> Modify by omitting the ball, or placing a light weight behind your knee.

>> Progress by lifting your supporting heel to relevé.

Side Lifts

This exercise focuses on the hip abductors, flexors, and extensors to develop trunk stabilization, improve hip flexor and extensor control, improve hip flexor and extensor flexion, and strengthen the hip abductors. Do 8 to 24 repetitions for each position. Get ready to lift and lower, go forward and back, around and up, and bend and extend!

Getting set

Stand tall, sideways to the barre, one arm's length away from the barre with your feet in a narrow first position. Place your inside forearm on the barre and your outside hand on your hip. Bend your knees slightly and lift your outside leg parallel to the floor (in line with your hip), as shown in Figure 8-17 (shown here with arm in high fifth as a progression).

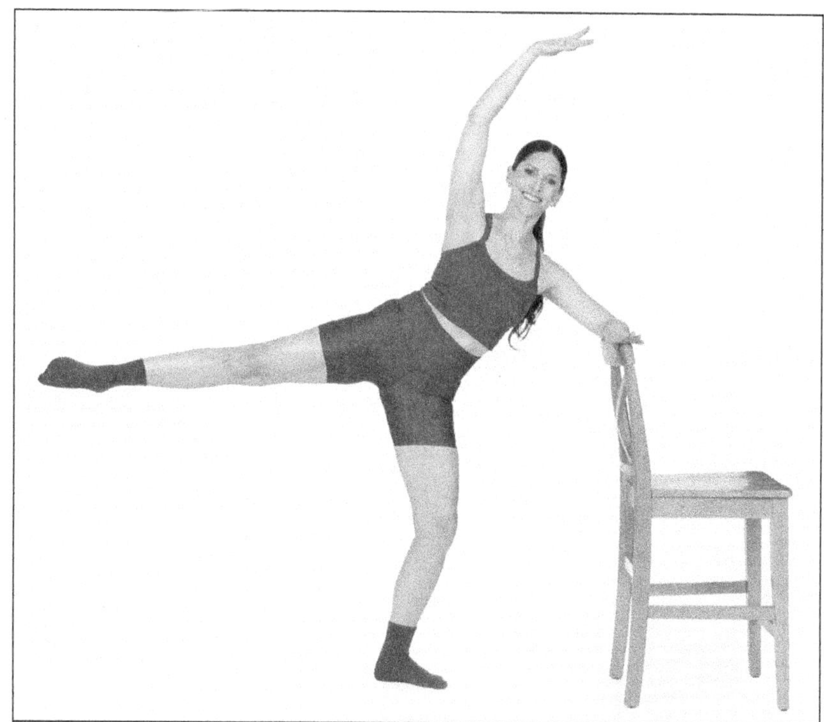

The movement

This movement involves three stages:

1. **Start with a lower and lift.**

   a. Begin by lifting your working leg a few inches from starting position and lowering it 1 inch, concentrating on the lift, not the lowering.

   b. Do 8 to 24 repetitions.

The straighter the leg, the more challenging the move is.

TIP

2. **Flow into bend and extend.**

   a. Bend your working leg slightly toward your body, and then stretch and extend.

   b. Squeeze your seat as you extend; the emphasis should be on the extension, not the bend.

   c. Do 8 to 24 repetitions.

3. **Flow into forward and back.**

   a. Lift your working leg and bring it to the front of your body.

   b. Lift your leg again to bring it toward the back of your body.

   c. Move your leg from front to back, with emphasis on lifting the whole leg to move it.

   d. Do 8 to 24 repetitions.

4. **Finish with circles.**

   a. Hold your working leg in line with your hip and begin to circle the leg in small motions; emphasis should be on lifting the leg as you circle it.

   b. Do 8 to 24 repetitions.

Finish with a relevé up and pivot to the barre.

Do's and don'ts

>> Do lift from under your waistline.

>> Do maintain a slight bend in the supporting leg.

>> Don't hyperextend.

>> Do keep your shoulders down and your abdominals in.

>> Do keep your head in line with your shoulders, hip, and foot.

The supportive leg should be mostly straight with a slight bend in the knee. Watch for hyperextension.

Variations

>> Modify by lowering the leg level and decreasing then number of repetitions.

>> Progress to perform each stage in relevé.

>> Transition: Face the barre on your other side or relevé up and pivot to the barre.

Resistance Band Series

The exercise focuses on the gluteus muscles and abductors to strengthen your hips and tone your seat and lower body. Do 8 slow repetitions or 16 fast in each direction. Grab your resistance band and weights and get ready to press and release.

Getting set

Stand tall at the barre facing forward or sideways. Stretch the band around your ankles. Stand with open legs to create tension on the band and soften both knees. Place weight on one leg and extend your other leg to the side. Straighten your working leg and flex the foot, making sure it is parallel and pointing forward, as shown in Figure 8-18.

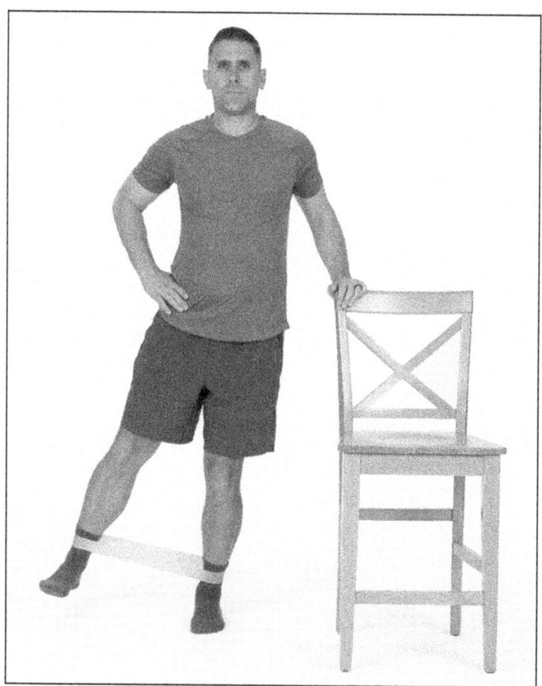

FIGURE 8-18: Place your weight on one leg and extend your other leg, making the band taut in your challenge zone.

The movement

This movement involves four stages:

1. **Start with an open/close.**

   a. Open one leg to the side as wide as possible, never releasing the resistance.

   b. Repeat 8 times slowly or 16 at tempo.

2. **Flow into circles.**

   a. Open one leg to the side as wide as possible, never releasing the resistance.

   b. Circle the leg with a small range of motion.

   c. Repeat 8 times slowly or 16 at tempo.

Keep your feet and legs parallel for stages 1 and 2.

3. **Flow into walks.**

   a. Keeping your feet parallel, side-walk out 2 counts and in 2 counts.

   b. Do 8 slow repetitions or 16 at tempo.

4. **Finish with cardio.**

   a. Chassé your inside foot four times toward the center of the room.

   b. Chassé your outside foot 4 times to return to the barre.

   c. Do eight to 24 repetitions.

A *chassé* is a simple traveling step where one foot steps out and the other foot quickly "chases" it to close the gap. Keep the movement light and controlled, stay low in your legs, and think smooth and rhythmic rather than big or bouncy.

Finish by removing the resistance band and standing tall.

Do's and don'ts

>> Do not lean into the supportive leg side.

>> Do keep your toes forward and flexed throughout the series.

>> Do engage your abdominals to support your back.

Variations

>> Modify by omitting the resistance band.

>> Progress in a relevé in the heel of the supporting leg.

>> Lift the opposite arm of the working leg high to create a lift in the side of the body.

Fold-Over Series

This exercise focuses on the gluteal muscles to strengthen the hip and tone the lower body. Do 8 to 16 repetitions for each position. Get ready to lift and lower.

Getting set

Stand facing the barre with your feet together in a parallel stance. Fold at your waist, placing your palms on the barre, as shown in Figure 8-19, or place folded arms on the barre with your head resting gently on your hands for extra support. Your heels should be directly under your hips, your toes under your navel, and your knees soft.

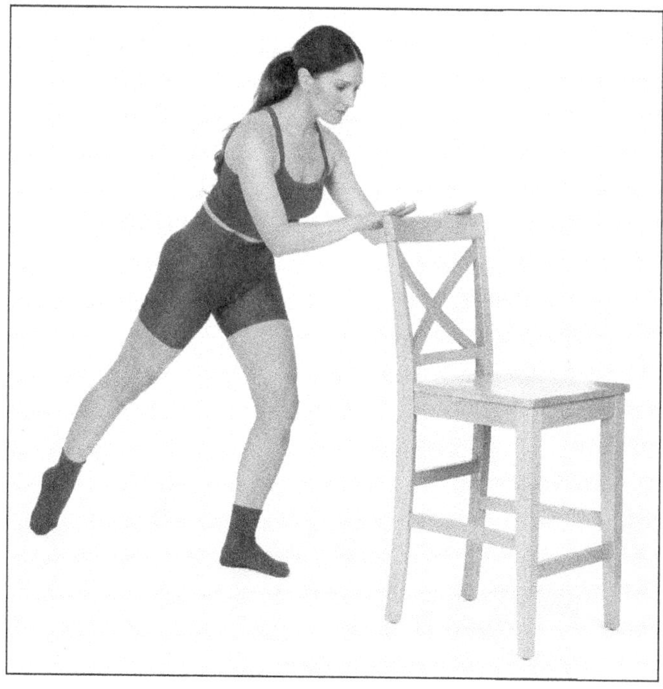

FIGURE 8-19: Start with your palms on the barre, ready to extend one leg back.

The movement

This movement has three stages:

1. **Start with a straight leg back.**

   a. Extend your leg parallel to the floor, straight behind your body, with a full range of motion (Figure 8-20).

   b. Do 8 repetitions.

   c. Pulse up with a pointed toe, then flex your foot and continue pulsing.

   d. Do 8 to 16 repetitions.

2. **Flow into a cross-back.**

   a. Cross the straight leg down to the floor and behind your supporting leg, and lift back up to parallel.

   b. Do 8 to 16 repetitions.

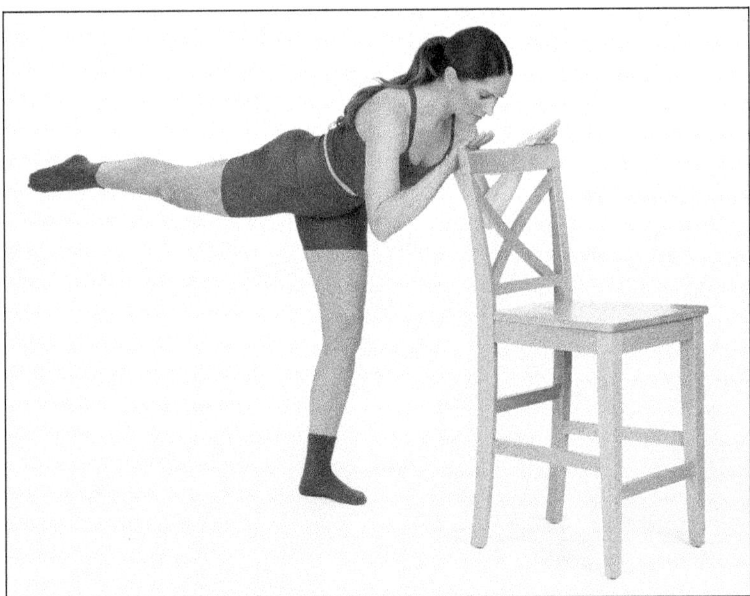

FIGURE 8-20: Extend your leg parallel to the floor.

3. **Finish with a hamstring curl.**

   a. Bend your knee so that the bottom of your foot is facing up.

   b. Move your foot down with a full range of motion.

   c. Do 8 repetitions.

   d. Pulse your foot up 8 to 16 times, activating your seat muscles.

   e. Point your toes and repeat.

Finish by stretching your seat.

Do's and don'ts

>> Do make sure your supportive leg remains bent throughout the series.

>> Do watch out for hyperextension and shoulder lifting.

>> Do keep your back straight, with no arching; activate your abdominals to protect your back.

>> Do keep the supportive leg mostly straight with a slight bend in the knee.

Variations

>> Modify by decreasing your range of motion.

>> Progress by extending your arms long on the barre, slightly wider than your shoulders.

>> Add circles to the back straight leg, bring your leg to the side as you lift it parallel to the floor, and/or perform each series with the supportive leg in relevé.

Chapter **9**

Strengthening Your Core

Time to get down on the mat! Strengthening your core is key to better posture, stability, and total-body strength, and in this chapter, I show you exactly how to do it the Barre way. Using small, precise movements, you target your powerhouse muscles from all angles, focusing on spinal and pelvic alignment and stability and building deep core engagement, all while holding, pulsing, and rotating in a C-curve — but feel free to place a ball at the base of your shoulder blades for extra support should you need it.

Exercises in This Chapter

The exercises in this chapter include the following:

» C-Curve Hold

» C-Curve Abs

» Supine Lifts

» Scissors

» Passé Abs

» Planking

For each exercise, I first help you prepare, and then I provide detailed steps for each one, followed by do's and don'ts to keep in mind as you practice. Finally, each section ends with ideas for variation.

You don't need much equipment for this chapter, but a good-quality exercise mat is essential to support your elbows, spine, and tailbone during floor work. A small ball is optional but helpful for added support in C-curve exercises, especially if you're building strength or protecting your lower back. Light hand weights are optional for progressions, but your own body weight is more than enough to get results here.

C-Curve Hold

Performed on the mat with your body in a C-like curve, this exercise strengthens your abdominal muscles and develops pelvic stability and control through tiny, focused movement. It's a small, simple movement with powerful results. Do 8 repetitions or pulses for each set.

Getting set

Get down on the mat and sit on your sit bones with your knees bent and relaxed, hip-distance apart, and your feet comfortably flat on the floor.

The movement

This movement has two stages — a hold and a series of small pulses.

1. **Start with a C-curve hold.**

   a. Lean on your forearms, keeping them flat on the floor, elbows in line with your shoulders, and palms facing down, to come up into a C-curve position (like a shallow sit-up), drawing your navel to your spine as your hips slightly tilt, with the back of your pelvis heavy into the floor (Figure 9-1).

   b. Slide your right arm down, and then your left arm down until you are resting on the pads of your elbows (keeping your elbows close to your ribcage), and your palms are facing up (Figure 9-2).

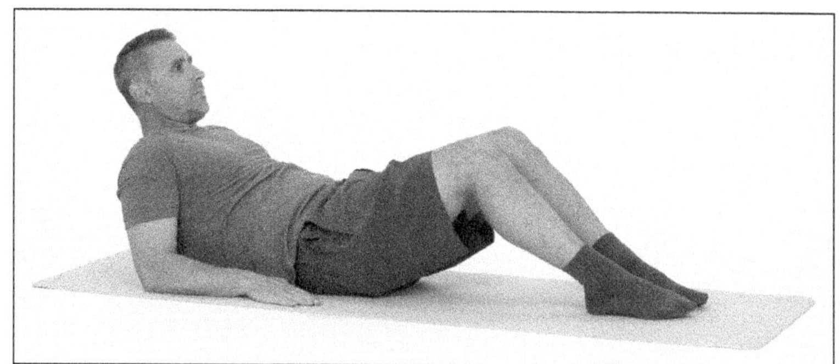

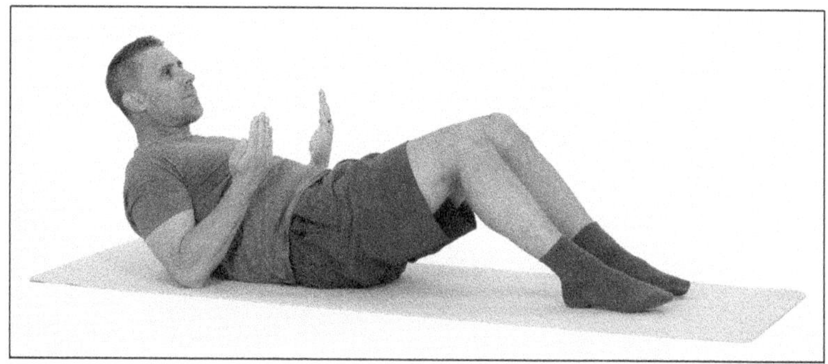

WARNING

Do not lean your weight onto the tip of the elbow and slide it away from your head to your hips.

    c. Keep your head up, neck relaxed, and your gaze pointed toward your knees.

    d. Hold for 8 counts for each set.

2. **Start the C-curve pulse.**

    a. From the C-curve hold in stage 1, begin to lift an inch, lower an inch, keeping your ribs next to your hips.

    b. Do 8 repetitions for each set.

Finish by rolling up to a seated position for C-curve abs.

Do's and don'ts

>> Do keep your sacrum anchored comfortably to the floor, releasing through your hip flexors.

>> Do maintain a neutral lumbar spine.

>> Do draw the base of your ribs to the back of your pelvis.

Variations

>> Modify by placing a ball at the base of your shoulder blades for support, and/or decrease your range of motion.

>> Progress by adding a small ball between your legs just above your knees for alignment with optional ball squeezes.

C-Curve Abs

Down on the mat with your body in a C-like curve, this exercise strengthens your abdominal muscles and develops pelvic stability and control through tiny, focused movements based around one position. Do 8 to 16 repetitions or counts for each set.

Getting set

Down on the mat, sit on your sit bones with your knees bent, hip distance apart, and feet comfortably flat on the floor.

TIP

Feel free to use a ball tucked into your lower back if you need a little extra support.

The movement

This movement involves seven stages:

1. **Start with C-curve abs.**

   a. Place your hands behind your thighs, just under your knees, to help guide you into a C-curve, rolling down to your challenge zone (Figure 9-3).

   b. Release your hands and hold for 8 to 16 counts.

2. **Add pulses down and up.**

   a. Curl the body down an inch, up an inch, keeping your ribs next to your hips.

   b. Repeat.

   c. Do 8 to 16 repetitions.

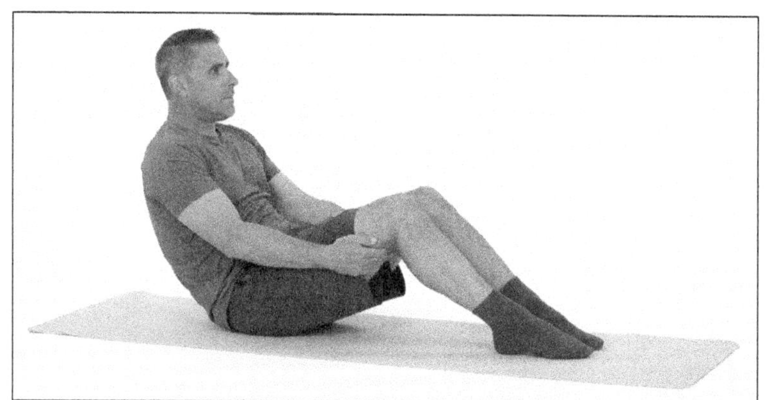

3. **Flow into arm rises.**

   a. Still in your challenge zone, put your arms in first position.

   b. Alternate lifting both arms to high fifth position.

   c. Go fast, then slow; you decide.

   d. Do 8 to 16 repetitions.

4. **Flow into paintbrush.**

   a. Still in your challenge zone, lift both arms up, leading with your wrists and your fingers pointing down (this will help slightly rotate the arm and wrists as you work, targeting small muscles).

   b. Lower your arms to the start position, leading with your wrists and your fingers pointing up, as if your hands are paintbrushes, painting a wall.

   c. Repeat.

   d. Do 8 to 16 repetitions.

5. **Flow into flexion and extension.**

   a. Still in your challenge zone, extend your arms forward, parallel to the floor, with your palms facing up.

   b. Flex at the elbows, performing a 90-degree bicep curl.

   c. Do 8 to 16 repetitions.

6. **Flow into arm circles.**

   a. Still in your challenge zone, extend your arms in front of your body and circle from the shoulders, no wider than shoulder width.

   b. Reverse direction. Keep your body still.

   c. Do 8 to 16 repetitions.

7. **Flow into oblique twists.**

    a. Still in your challenge zone, extend your arms forward with your palms facing down.

    b. Rotate your ribcage to the right (Figure 9-4).

    c. Curl down an inch, up an inch, maintaining rotation of your torso.

        Option 1: Add fist taps by lightly bumping your fists together.

        Option 2: Extend your right leg to 45 degrees. Hold the position for 8 counts, and then tap your fists together.

    d. Rotate back to center, and repeat on your left side.

    e. Do 8 to 16 repetitions.

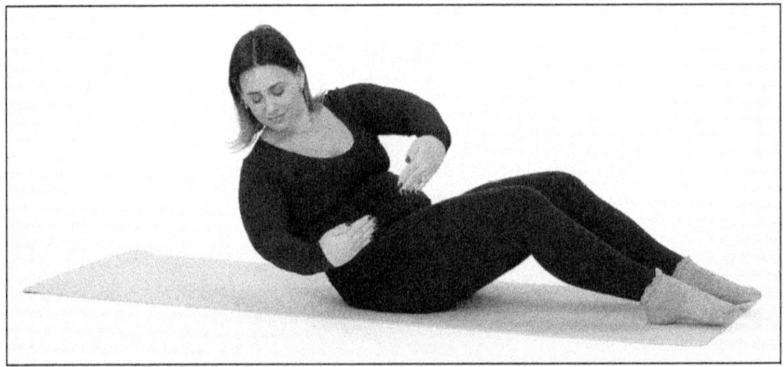

FIGURE 9-4: Rotate your ribcage and curl up and down an inch.

Finish by sitting tall or lying down.

Do's and don'ts

>> Do keep your abdominals anchored while your extremities are moving.

>> Do remain in your challenge zone throughout the variations.

>> Do maintain rib-to-hip connection through the front line of your abdominals to stop you from engaging your lower back.

>> Do keep your collarbones spread and your shoulder blades "seat-belted" across your back.

Variations

>> If you have lower-back issues or weak lower abdominals, use a ball behind your spine for tactile support, and/or decrease your range of motion.

>> Progress by adding a small ball between your legs just above your knees for alignment, and add in optional ball squeezes, and/or add light arm weights.

Supine Lifts

Performed on the mat with your body lying flat and relaxed in the supine position, this exercise strengthens your abdominal muscles and develops pelvic stability and control through tiny, focused movement. Do 8 repetitions for each set.

Getting set

Lie supine with your legs extended long on the mat. Use your hands to cup the base of your skull; keep your elbows out. Cross one ankle over the other and softly point your toes, as shown in Figure 9-5.

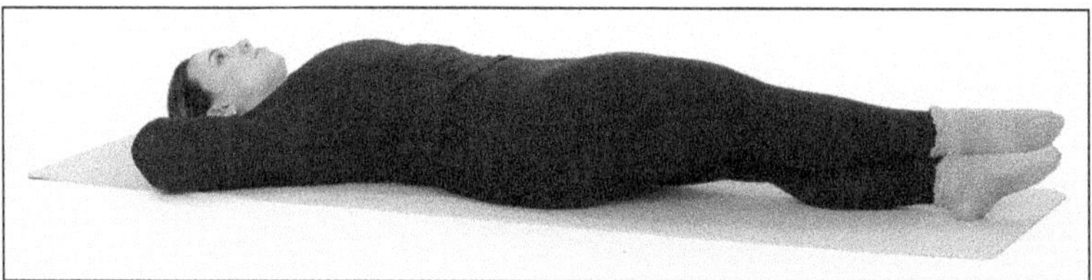

FIGURE 9-5: The starting position for supine lifts.

The movement

This movement involves four stages:

1. **Start with a lift and lower.**

    a. Curl your abdominals using a forward contraction, allowing your head, neck, and shoulders to rise from the mat and into your challenge zone. Keep your eyeline toward your toes (Figure 9-6).

    b. Return to the start position.

    c. Do 8 repetitions.

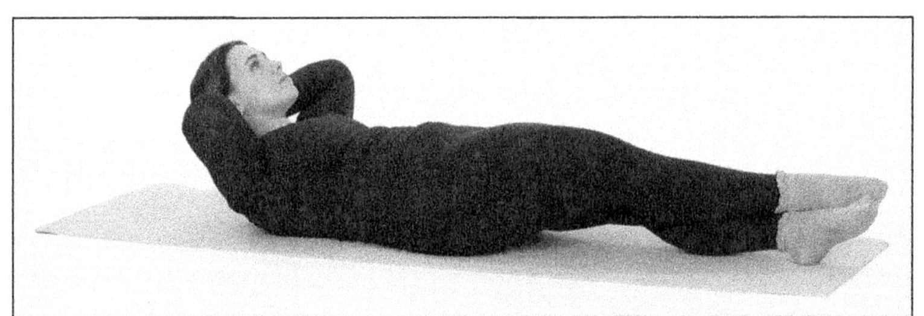

2. **Flow into inches.**

   a. Curl your abdominals again as in stage 1, and slowly and mindfully curl up an inch, then down an inch, keeping your ribs next to your hips.

      Option: Increase the tempo to tiny pulses.

   b. Do 8 repetitions.

3. **Maintaining your C-curve, flow into a single-leg tabletop/straight leg.**

   a. Maintaining your forward contraction, draw one leg into a tabletop position, keeping your calf parallel to the mat.

   b. Pulse that thigh to your chest.

   c. Pulse your chest to your thigh.

   d. Then, do both moves simultaneously, pulsing your chest to your thigh and thigh to chest.

   e. Next, extend your working leg to the ceiling and repeat your pulses.

   f. Repeat on the other side.

   g. Do 8 repetitions for each set.

This series can be broken down into individual elements, as required.

TIP

4. **Maintaining your C-curve, flow into a single-leg tabletop rotation.**

   a. Maintain your forward contraction and draw one leg into a tabletop position, keeping your calf parallel with the mat.

   b. Rotate your torso toward your lifted leg.

   c. Rotate back to center and repeat. Play with tempo, go fast or slow; you decide, but maintain forward contraction throughout.

   d. Repeat on the other side.

   e. Do 8 repetitions for each set.

Finish by extending your legs and lowering your head to set up for the next exercise.

Do's and don'ts

» Do hold your chest proud and your neck relaxed, and be mindful of pulling on the back of your head.

» Do anchor from your abdominals. Think: ribs to hips.

» Do support your lower back by drawing your naval to your spine.

» Do keep your elbows in your peripheral vision.

Variations

» Modify by performing this series with your knees bent and your feet flat on the floor.

» Progress by floating your bottom leg 1 inch off the mat.

Scissors

Like the previous supine lifts, this exercise has you lying down on the mat, your body in the supine position — flat and relaxed. You'll scissor your legs to strengthen your abdominal muscles and develop pelvic lumbar stability and control through focused movement. Although you'll be increasing hamstring and hip flexor flexibility, this movement should be powered by your abs as much as possible. Do 8 to 16 repetitions for each set.

Getting set

Lie supine with your knees bent and your feet flat on the floor. Lift your legs to a tabletop position, then extend them to the ceiling, keeping your legs and feet in either parallel or external rotation. Your hands should be down by your side, or contract your abs forward with your hands at the base of your skull.

Support your neck with your hands whenever you feel the need — your neck should always stay relaxed.

The movement

This movement involves three stages:

1. **Start with a single-leg scissor.**

   a. Draw your left leg toward your torso and lower your right leg to your challenge zone (without touching the mat).

   b. Place both hands behind your left calf and bend your elbows.

   c. Pulse your upper body toward your leg for one set (Figure 9-7).

   d. Then, place your hands gently behind your head and engage your abs to pulse your leg toward your torso for one set.

   e. Pulse your leg and torso toward each other at the same time for one set.

   f. Repeat on the other side.

   g. Do 8 to 16 repetitions for each set.

2. **Flow into a scissor crisscross.**

   a. Rotate your torso toward your lifted leg and return to center as your legs pass one another, one lowering, one raising up.

   b. Repeat on the other side and continue alternating.

   c. Do 8 to 16 repetitions for each set.

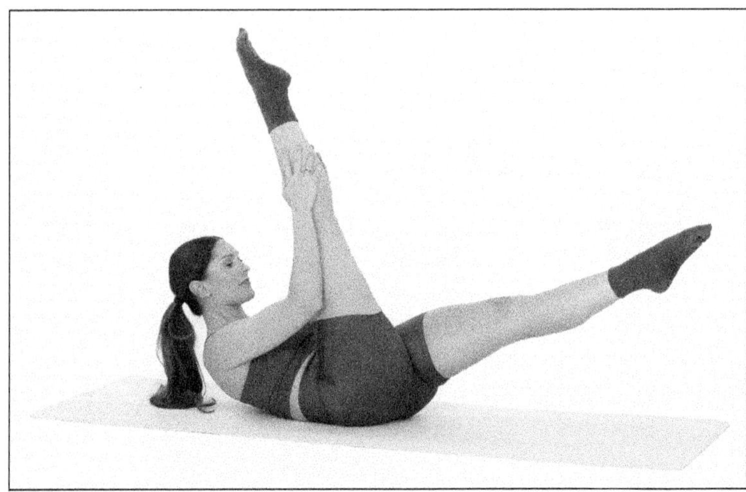

FIGURE 9-7: Pulse your leg toward your torso.

3. **Finally, flow into a stuck scissor.**

    a. Extend your legs to a scissor position with one leg raised high and one lower (off the mat) and draw your whole shape toward your torso and lower, maintaining distance between your legs.

    b. Add a torso rotation (Figure 9-8).

    c. Repeat on the other side.

    d. Do 8 to 16 repetitions for each set.

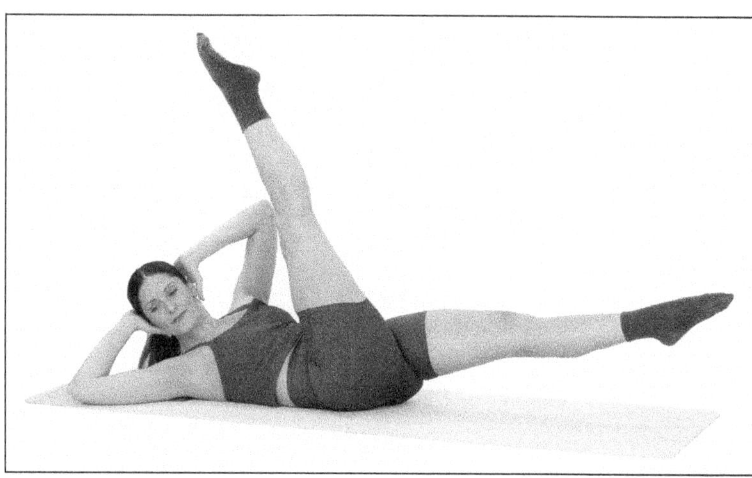

FIGURE 9-8: Add a torso rotation.

Finish by extending your legs and lowering your head to set up for the next series.

Do's and don'ts

» Don't allow hyperflexion of the neck and weight-loading on the cervical spine.

» Don't allow your hip flexors to take over.

» Do maintain stability when performing the scissoring movement.

» Do keep your navel to your spine.

» Do keep the back of your pelvis anchored to the mat.

Variations

>> Modify by softening your knees to reduce the length of the lever.

>> Progress by flowing from one movement to the next, maintaining forward contraction.

Passé Abs

Performed down on the mat, sitting on your sit bones, this abs exercise strengthens your abdominal muscles and develops pelvic lumbar stability and control through focused movement. Do 8 repetitions for each set (up to 2 sets).

Getting set

Roll down and sit up on the mat. Lean back to rest on your forearms, keeping your elbows in line with your shoulders and your head, neck, and shoulders raised. Draw your legs to a tabletop position. Extend your left leg long and place the arch of your right foot glued to the inside of the left knee, as shown in Figure 9-9, and your right knee close to your midline (in a parallel passé).

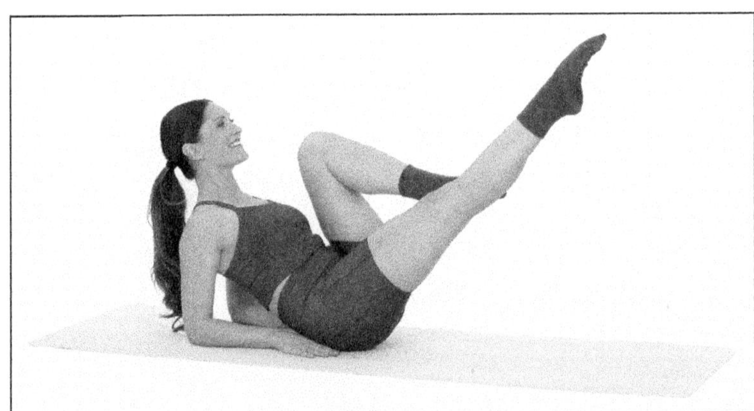

FIGURE 9-9: Place the arch of your right foot glued to the inside of the left knee.

The movement

This movement involves four stages:

1. **Start with passé abs, parallel.**

   a. Lower your legs away from your body to your challenge zone.

   b. Return to the start position.

   c. Repeat.

   d. Then, switch legs, passing through a tabletop position to maintain form.

   e. Do 8 repetitions for each set (up to 2 sets).

2. **Flow into turned-out passé abs.**

   a. Repeat the series as in stage 1, but with your bent leg in an external rotation.

   b. Do 8 repetitions for each set (up to 2 sets).

3. **Flow into a sweep.**

   a. From your turned-out position (stage 2), lower your legs to your challenge zone and draw them toward your right shoulder.

   b. Sweep through to the start position.

   c. Then, sweep your legs toward your left shoulder.

   d. Repeat.

   e. Do 8 repetitions for each set (up to 2 sets). Then swap your legs and repeat.

4. **Finish with an extend.**

   a. With control, slide your foot down your leg to meet the other foot (Figure 9-10).

   b. Return to the start position. Repeat on both sides.

   c. Do 8 repetitions for each set (up to 2 sets).

Finish by lengthening your legs to set up the next exercise.

Do's and don'ts

>> Do maintain pelvic alignment throughout.

>> Do keep your tailbone and sacrum anchored.

>> Do focus on the "lift" of the action.

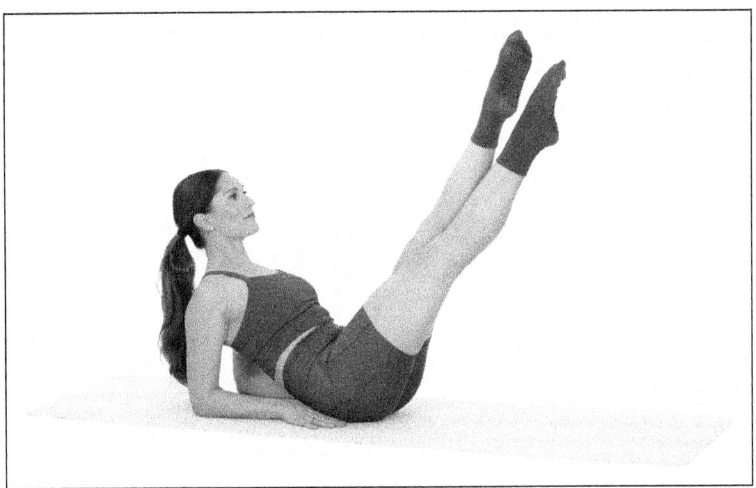

Variations

» Modify by reducing your range of motion, the number of repetitions, and/or performing in coupé instead of passé.

» Progress by flowing from one set to the next, increasing your range of motion, and/or the number of repetitions.

TECHNICAL STUFF

Performing in *coupé* means your foot rests lightly at the ankle instead of higher up the leg. It's a shorter lever, better balance, and a great way to keep the work strong without wobbling all over the place.

Planking

The plank is a classic exercise for a reason: The intense hold activates your core muscles and so much more. This version — with a series of Barre moves — focuses on the upper body and abdominals, and can fully fatigue your body. (Cue the "Barre shakes"!) For this exercise, you'll be on the mat, doing 4 repetitions on each side for a total of 8 repetitions.

Getting set

Start in a quadruped position on all fours with your forearms and palms on the floor. Slide your knees back until your upper body is in a modified plank position, with your forearms and hands slightly wider than your shoulders, and your pelvis slightly tilted forward.

The movement

This movement has six stages:

1. **Start with a classic plank.**

   a. Tuck your toes under and lengthen your legs into a full plank position, knees off the mat.

   b. Keep your hands directly under your shoulders, your neck in line with your spine and relaxed, and maintain a long line from the crown of your head to your toes (Figure 9-11).

   c. Hold for 8 counts.

2. **Flow into a relevé series.**

   a. Rock forward onto your toes and back to your heels, articulating your feet as your weight shifts front to back.

   b. Do 4 or 8 repetitions.

3. **Then, dip your hips.**

   a. In your plank stance, gently dip your right hip toward the floor and lift through your center to dip your left hip to the floor, moving fluidly from right to left, maintaining the connection of your ankles and inner thighs.

   b. Do 4 or 8 repetitions on each side.

4. **Flow into a passé series.**

   a. Make a slight external rotation of the legs to bring your feet into a Pilates "V" (heels together, toes apart).

   b. Draw your right leg to passé (Figure 9-12).

   c. Return to the start position.

   d. Repeat on the other leg.

   e. Do 4 or 8 repetitions on each side.

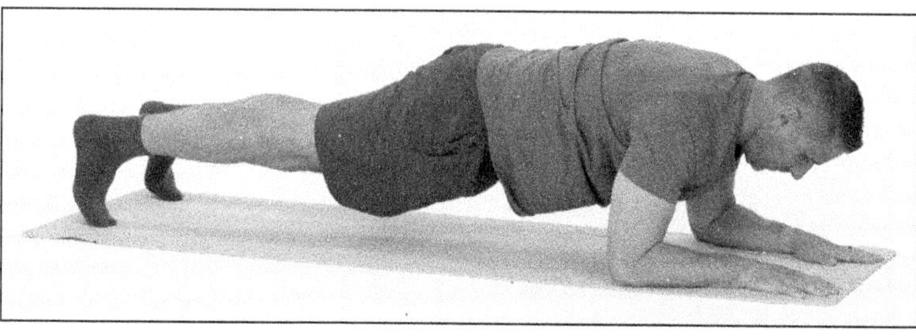

FIGURE 9-11: The classic plank position (shown here with elbows on the mat).

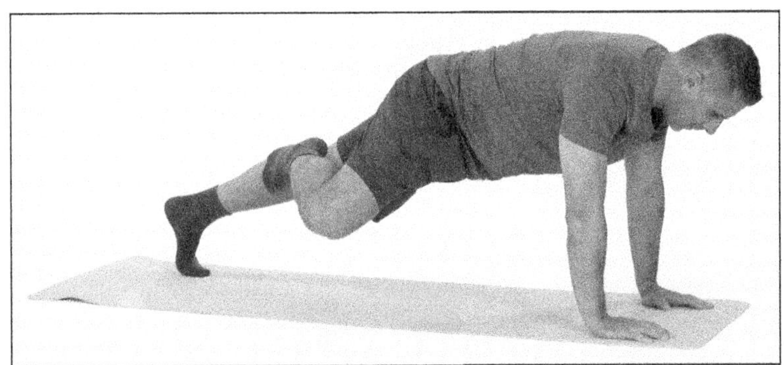

5. **Then, développé.**

   a. Extend your leg from passé to a side extension. Hold the extension and close back to the start position.

   b. Repeat on your left leg. The cue here is: "Passé, développé, hold, close."

   c. Do 4 or 8 repetitions on each side.

6. **Finish with a combo.**

   a. Combine the relevé and single passé in slight external rotation, alternating sides.

   b. Do 4 or 8 repetitions on each side.

Finish by pressing back into an active rest stretch, then follow with upper-body stretches.

Do's and don'ts

» Do maintain a neutral spine with a strong abdominal connection. There should be no lower back pain or discomfort at all.

» Do maintain your pubic bone to your navel.

» Do start with a slow tempo before lifting to a quicker tempo.

» Do create a long line from your tailbone to the crown of your head.

Variations

» Modify by remaining in a modified plank position throughout and/or take a break between sets.

» Progress by increasing the number of repetitions with no breaks between sets.

Chapter **10**

Firing Up Your Lower Body

This chapter presents a lower-body set to fire up your glutes, hips, and thighs with focused, floor-based movements.

Exercises in This Chapter

The exercises in this chapter include the following:

» Side-Seat Series

» Love to Hate

» Bottoms Up

For each exercise, I first help you prepare, and then I provide detailed steps for each one, followed by do's and don'ts to keep in mind as you practice. Finally, each section ends with ideas for variation.

To complete the first set of exercises in this chapter, first, roll out your mat and grab a stretch (or resistance) band. Because stretch bands come in several different strengths, make sure the resistance you choose is strong enough to put you into your challenge zone.

Side-Seat Series

This side-lying sequence works your glutes, hip flexors, and hamstrings while strengthening your pelvic and lumbar stability. These exercises help you improve hip control, flexibility, and the ability to move one leg independently of the other while keeping your body still — a key element of Barre technique.

Getting set

Place a stretch band around your thighs just above your knees. Lie on your side with your knees bent at a 90-degree angle so that your knees line up with your hips. Keep your feet in line with your knees. Rest your bottom arm long or folded under your head and place your top hand lightly on the mat in front of your torso for support.

The movement

The movement involves two main actions: Lift and lower and the clam. Follow each action and its variation for 8 to 16 repetitions per position. This series builds in simple phases to help you strengthen and mobilize your hip while maintaining stable alignment.

1. **Start with lift and lower.**

   a. Lift your top leg off your bottom leg while keeping it parallel to the floor (Figure 10-1).

   b. Flow back down to your starting position, maintaining firm contact with the floor with your supporting leg.

   c. Repeat for the full count.

Think of lifting your leg from the crease of your hip rather than from your knee to target your seat more effectively.

2. **Move into the first variation: Knee to toe.**

   a. Lift your top leg parallel to the mat.

   b. Internally rotate your thigh bone so that your knees touch.

   c. Return to parallel, pressing gently into the band.

   d. Externally rotate your thigh bone so that your toes touch (Figure 10-2).

   e. Repeat, working to keep your top leg lifted the entire time.

Keep your pelvis steady. Your thigh rotates, but your hips should stay stacked like two blocks.

3. **Move into the second variation: Lift and pulse (parallel).**

   a. Lift your top leg again (Figure 10-1) and draw your thigh bone slightly toward your chest while staying parallel to the floor.

   b. Begin pulsing upward with a controlled tempo.

   c. Increase the tempo once you feel the muscles activate deeply.

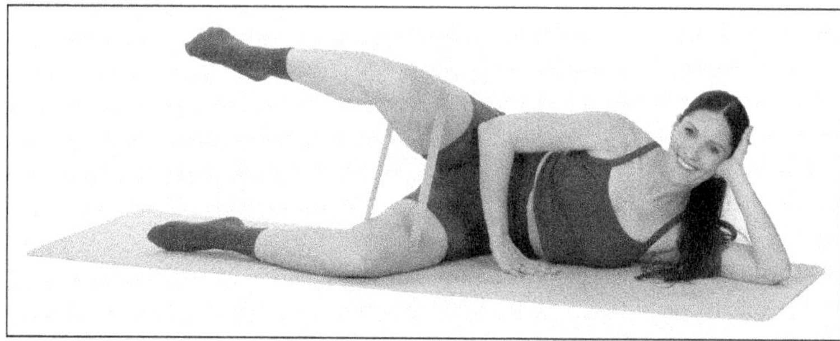

FIGURE 10-1: Lift your top leg off your bottom leg while keeping it parallel to the floor.

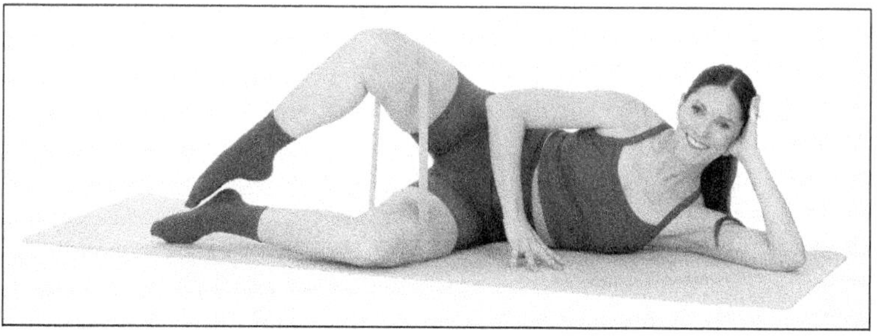

FIGURE 10-2: Externally rotate your thigh bone so that your toes touch.

4. **Then, flow into the clam.**

   a. Keep your feet glued together as you open your knees apart, as shown in Figure 10-3 (shown here raised up on the lower forearm as an advanced option).

   b. Pause briefly at the top of the movement.

   c. Slowly resist your knees back to the starting position.

   d. Repeat for the full count.

5. **End with the elevated clam variation.**

   a. Keep your feet together and lift them off the mat to hip height (Figure 10-4).

   b. Open your top knee away from your bottom knee (Figure 10-5).

   c. Pause at the top, then resist the closing motion with control.

   d. Repeat.

   e. Repeat the entire series on the other side.

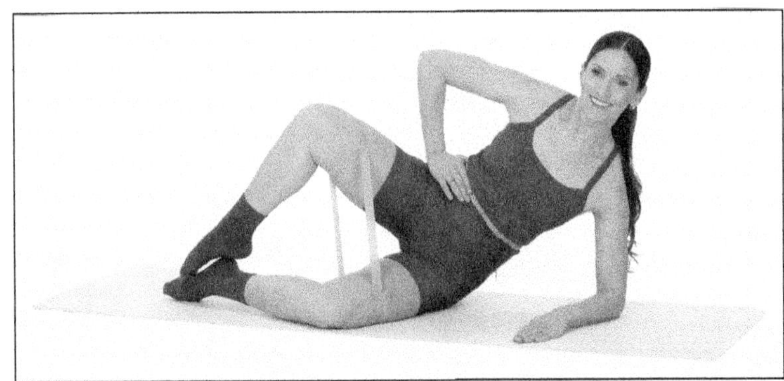

FIGURE 10-3: Keep your feet glued together as you open your knees apart.

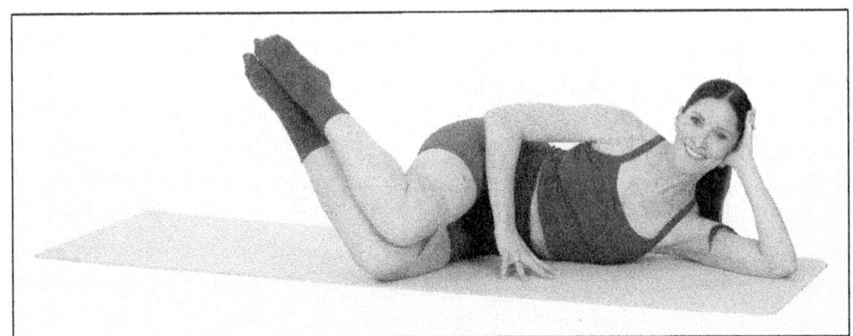

FIGURE 10-4: Keep your feet together and lift them off the mat to hip height.

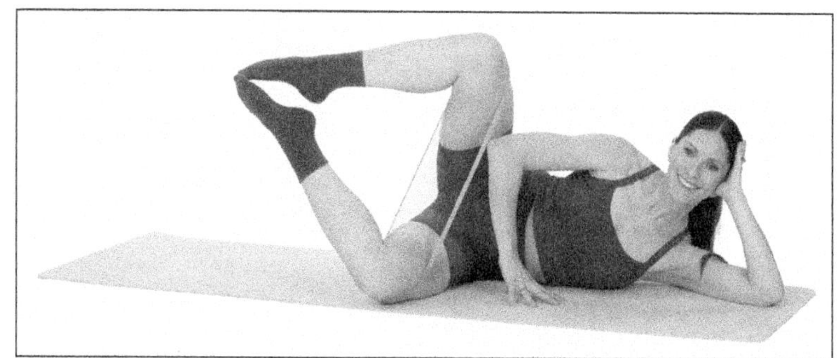

Keep scooping your bottom waistline away from the floor to prevent collapse and keep your hips aligned.

The side-seat series is an excellent strengthening and mobility series before stretching your hips or moving on to standing seat work. Notice how your hips feel more stable and supported after completing both sides.

Do's and don'ts

>> Do keep your hips and shoulders stacked vertically.

>> Do lift your bottom waistline away from the mat to avoid sinking.

>> Do keep your top shoulder relaxed and away from your ear.

>> Don't swing your leg or let momentum take over; small, controlled movements work best.

Variations

>> Modify by removing the resistance band or reducing your range of motion.

>> Reduce the number of repetitions if your hips fatigue quickly.

>> Progress by placing your top arm behind your head to decrease external support and increase core demand.

>> Progress by raising up onto your forearm for elevated clams (Figure 10-6).

>> Try straightening your top leg during the lift and lower series to add lever length and intensify the challenge.

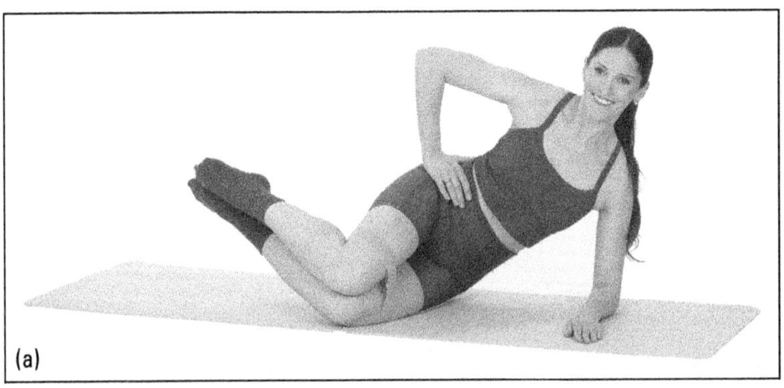

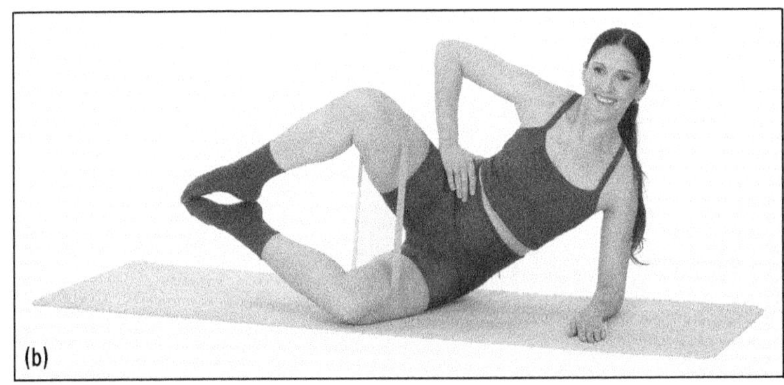

FIGURE 10-6: On your forearm, keep your feet together and lift them off the mat to hip height (a), then open your top knee away from your bottom knee (b).

Love to Hate

This targeted, side-lying series strengthens your glutes, hip flexors, and hamstrings while improving pelvic–lumbar stability, hip mobility, and leg independence. Expect a deep burn. (This one really earns its name!)

Getting set

Lie on your side with your legs extended together in parallel, forming an "L" shape. Flex your feet and keep them in line with your hips. Rest your bottom arm long or folded under your head and place your top hand on the floor in front of your torso for support.

The movement

Follow each action and variation for 8 to 16 repetitions. This series builds through simple, precise motions that help you strengthen your hips while keeping your pelvis steady.

1. **Start with lift and lower.**

    a. Lift your top leg off your bottom leg, keeping it parallel to the floor.

    b. Pulse your thigh bone upward in small, controlled movements.

    c. Repeat for the full count.

Keep your foot flexed and your leg long. This helps activate your outer hip muscles more deeply.

2. **Move into the first variation: Internal rotation.**

    a. Lift your top leg to parallel.

    b. Internally rotate your thigh bone so that your toes lightly touch your bottom foot.

    c. Return to parallel with control.

    d. Repeat for the full count.

Your thigh rotates, not your hip. Keep your pelvis perfectly still.

3. **Move into the second variation: The front/back sweep.**

    a. Lift your top leg to parallel.

    b. Gently swing your leg forward a few inches.

    c. Bring it back just past your hip line without arching your lower back.

    d. Repeat with smooth, even pacing.

4. **End with the final variation: The rainbow tap.**

    a. Lift your top leg to parallel.

    b. Draw a small rainbow shape with your foot, tapping gently in front of you and behind you.

    c. Keep the movement light, lifted, and controlled.

    d. Repeat the entire series on your opposite side.

Imagine your toes tracing a tiny semicircle in the air. Height doesn't matter as much as control.

After completing both sides, lie on your back to stretch through your hips and outer thighs. Your glutes have worked hard — this ending helps you restore length and ease.

Do's and don'ts

>> Do keep your hips and shoulders stacked.

>> Do scoop the side of your torso up and away from the mat.

>> Do keep your top shoulder relaxed.

>> Don't drop your leg; lower it with slow, deliberate resistance.

Variations

>> Modify by reducing your range of motion or decreasing the number of repetitions.

>> Progress by increasing the number of repetitions while maintaining clean alignment.

>> Try extending your top leg fully during the front and back sweep or rainbow variations for an added challenge.

>> Add a light ankle weight only once you can maintain proper form.

Bottoms Up

This bridge-based series strengthens your glutes, hamstrings, hips, and core while helping you build pelvic–lumbar stability. You'll also develop control through your abdominals and hamstrings as you articulate your spine through each repetition. I offer several choices for your single-leg exercises in this series; only attempt one or two of these, as doing them all proves too intense.

Getting set

Lie on your back with your knees bent and your feet on the floor. Extend your arms long by your sides with your fingertips reaching toward your heels. Relax your head, neck, and shoulders into the mat.

The movement

Work through the sequence using 16 repetitions for each set. This series builds upward from a basic bridge to progressively more challenging variations that are all designed to help you activate your posterior chain with precision.

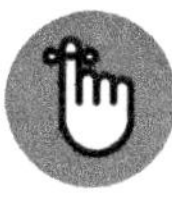

Choose only one or two of the following movements.

1. Start with the first action: Lift and pulse.

   a. Press into your feet and articulate your spine as you lift into a high bridge (Figure 10-7).

   b. Lower back to the mat by articulating your spine down one vertebra at a time.

   c. Repeat for the full set.

   d. On the final repetition, hold at the top and lower your hips down an inch, then up an inch to "pulse" the movement.

   e. Repeat to maintain small, controlled pulses.

Think of sending your knees forward as you lift — this helps activate your glutes rather than your lower back.

2. Choose Option 1: Single-leg lift and pulse.

   a. From your high bridge, float your right leg into a tabletop position.

   b. Perform the same lift and pulse pattern while keeping your hips level.

   c. Maintain even weight through your supporting foot.

Think of your pelvis as a "tabletop" — it shouldn't tip when the leg lifts.

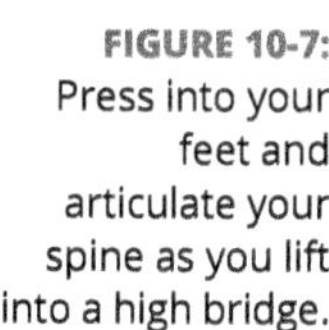

FIGURE 10-7: Press into your feet and articulate your spine as you lift into a high bridge.

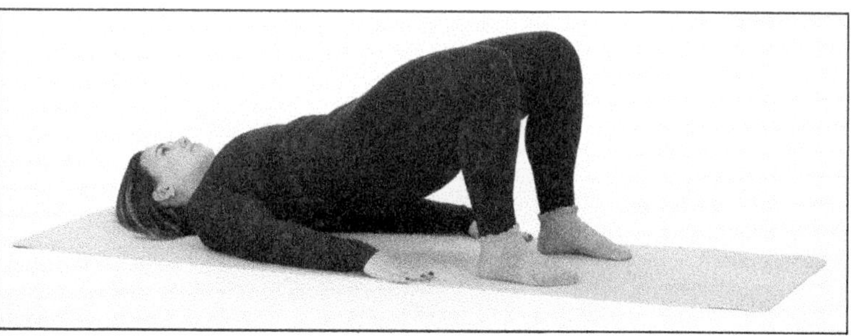

3. **Or choose Option 2: Paintbrush.**

   a. Begin in your single-leg tabletop position.

   b. Extend your working leg straight toward the ceiling.

   c. Point your foot as you lengthen upward (Figure 10-8).

   d. Flex your foot as you lower your straight leg down (as if your foot is a paintbrush, painting a wall).

   e. Point your toes again as you lift your leg back to the starting position.

   f. Repeat, keeping your hips lifted and stable throughout.

4. **Progress to the final action: Open and close.**

   a. Lift into a high bridge using full spinal articulation.

   b. Extend one leg straight toward the ceiling and flex your foot.

   c. Open your lifted leg outward from your centerline while maintaining pelvic stability.

   d. Return to center with control.

   e. Repeat for the full set.

   f. Repeat the entire series on your opposite side.

If your hips begin to drop or twist, reduce the size of your leg movement to maintain stability.

TIP

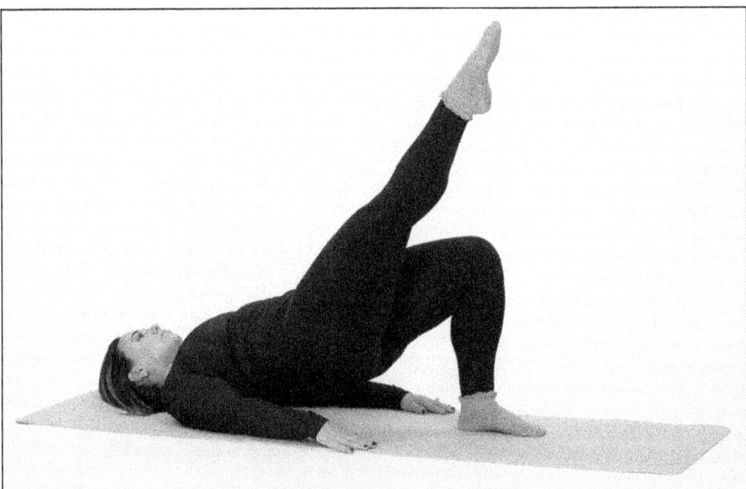

FIGURE 10-8: Point your foot as you lengthen up.

After completing both sides, hug your knees into your chest to release your lower back and gently transition into your cooldown stretches.

Do's and don'ts

» Do keep your arms long by your sides with your fingertips reaching toward your toes.

» Do relax your head, neck, and shoulders throughout the sequence.

» Don't thrust your ribs upward. Keep them softly knit to support spinal articulation.

» Don't rush the lowering phase; articulate slowly for greater control.

Variations

» Modify by keeping both feet on the floor throughout.

» Reduce your range of motion or decrease the number of repetitions if your lower back or hamstrings fatigue.

» Progress by placing light weights on your hips or lifting your arms toward the ceiling to challenge stability.

» Try holding at the top of the bridge for a longer endurance challenge.

Chapter **11**

Active Stretching

Active stretching is where the magic happens. Stretching helps your muscles recover, improves your flexibility, and leaves you feeling recharged. I suggest adding stretching to your daily routine. Why? Because it truly improves your flexibility and mobility if done consistently. In short, I'm a big stretch fan! This chapter guides you through full-body stretches inspired by functional movement.

Stretches in This Chapter

The stretches in this chapter include the following:

» Upper-Body Stretch Series

» Seat Stretches

» Abs and Torso Stretch Series

» Full-Body Ballet Stretches

» Floor Stretches

» Balance Ending

Upper-Body Stretch Series

This upper-body stretch sequence helps you improve flexibility, prevent soreness, reduce your risk of injury, and reset your posture before moving on to Barre work. These stretches target your shoulders, triceps, chest, wrists, and sides to help you release tension from upper-body strengthening exercises.

Getting set

You can perform this series while sitting or standing in the center of the floor. Choose whichever position allows you to sit or stand tall with your ribs relaxed and your shoulders down.

The movement

Work through the following five stretches, holding each for 16 to 32 counts. Rest halfway through if needed. This sequence unfolds through simple stretches designed to lengthen your upper body safely.

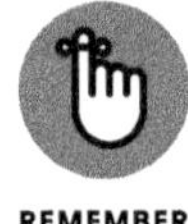

Do this stretch series *immediately* after all your upper-body strength work and before the Barre section. This helps restore muscle balance, improves posture, and prepares your body for standing exercises — and feels great.

Arm crossover

1. Lift one arm in front of your chest and draw it across your midline.

2. Hook your opposite arm underneath to support and deepen the stretch (Figure 11-1).

3. Gently press both arms into one another to find active resistance while keeping your shoulders down.

4. Repeat on the other side.

Keep your shoulders "melting" down your back; this instantly increases effectiveness.

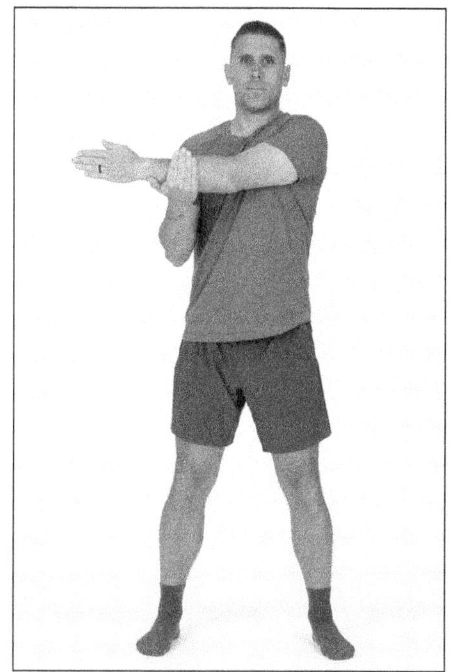

Triceps stretch

1. Reach one arm overhead toward the ceiling.

2. Bend your elbow so your fingertips point down your upper back.

3. Place your opposite hand on your bent elbow and apply gentle pressure.

4. Resist the elbow and hand into one another to activate the stretch.

5. Repeat on the other side.

Avoid letting your ribs flare; it's a triceps stretch, not a backbend.

Chest expansion with fold-over

1. Stand or sit tall with your feet together.

2. Interlace your fingers behind your back and draw your shoulders downward.

3. Connect the heels of your hands and lengthen your arms.

4. Fold forward from your waist, lowering your chest while lifting your hands behind you (Figure 11-2).

5. Maintain a long spine as you open your chest and shoulders.

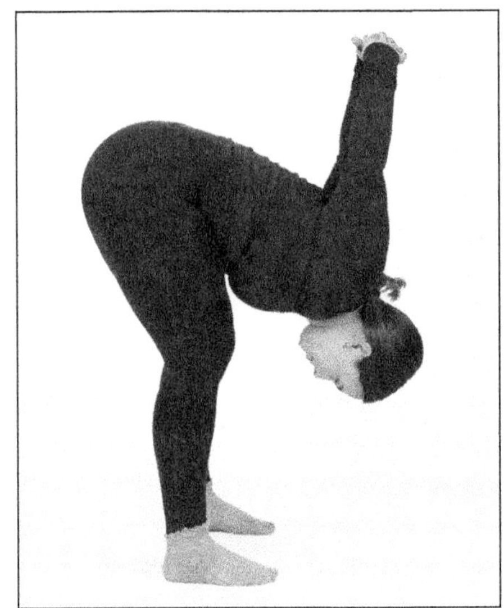

TIP

Keep your collarbones broad so the stretch travels across the entire front of your body.

Wrist connect

1. Lift both arms overhead.

2. Hold one wrist with the opposite hand.

3. Lengthen upward through your torso, then gently pull your wrist sideways to open your arm and waist (Figure 11-3).

4. Repeat on the other side.

Side reach on floor

1. Sit comfortably on the mat with your sit bones anchored.

2. Reach one arm overhead.

3. Laterally flex to the side, keeping both hips grounded (Figure 11-4).

4. Repeat on both sides.

TIP

Visualize space opening between each rib to create length, not collapse.

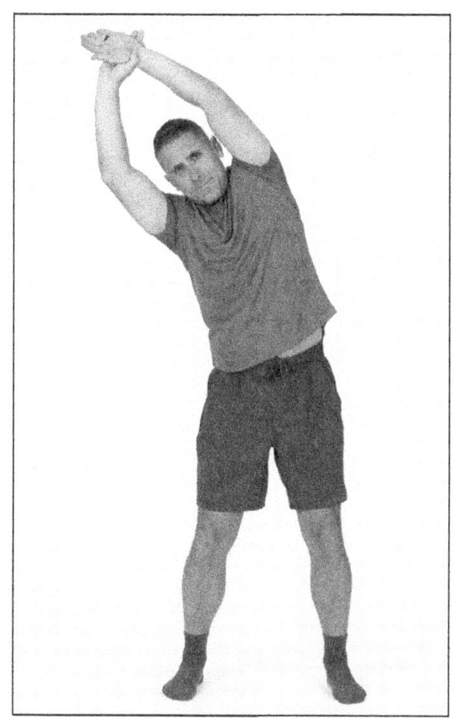

FIGURE 11-3:
Gently pull your
wrist sideways,
lengthening
through
your torso.

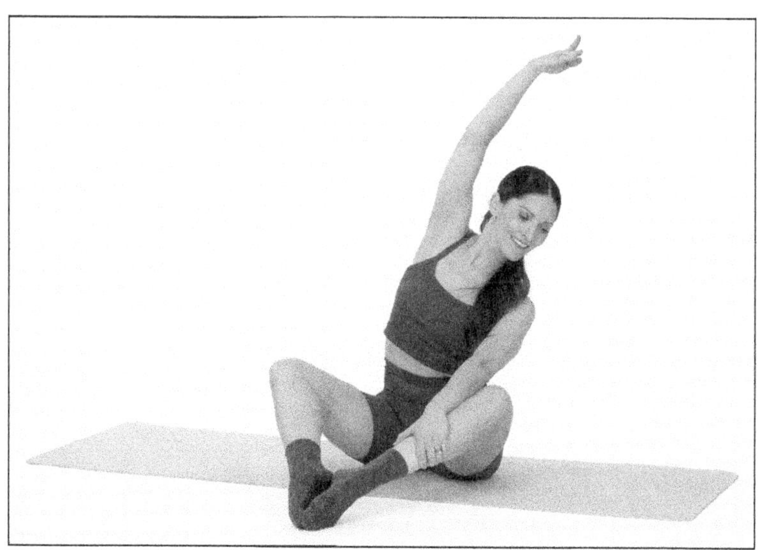

FIGURE 11-4:
Flex to one side,
reaching your
arm overhead.

Do's and don'ts

>> Do hold each stretch for 16 counts and split into two sets of 8 if needed.

>> Do keep your shoulders down for the initial stretch and your rib cage relaxed.

>> Do keep your hips and shoulders square in every position.

>> Don't rush; use breath, control, and alignment to deepen each stretch safely.

Variations

>> Decrease your range of motion if you feel discomfort or have limited flexibility.

>> Increase your range of motion gradually as your body warms and flexibility improves.

Seat Stretches

This stretch series targets your glutes and hamstrings to improve flexibility, reduce soreness, and support strong, efficient movement during seat work — and a little sassy walk. You'll feel sassy when you do it!

Use these stretches after your seat section to release tension in your hips, glutes, and hamstrings. They're especially effective when your muscles are warm and ready to lengthen.

Getting set

Stand at a countertop, sturdy chair, or table. You'll use only light fingertip support for balance. Keep your spine long and your abs gently engaged.

The movement

Work through the following four stretches, holding each for 16 to 32 counts. This series moves through simple positions that help you safely release your seat and hamstrings.

Pretzel stretch (standing figure-four)

1. Stand tall with your feet together, lightly holding onto a countertop or chairback for balance if needed.
2. Cross one ankle over the opposite thigh to form a figure-four position.
3. Bend your supporting knee into a soft plié.
4. Flex your lifted foot to protect your knee.
5. Fold forward slightly from your waist to deepen the stretch.
6. Repeat on the other side.

Imagine moving your hips straight back, as if you're about to sit down, not twisting. This helps target your glutes evenly.

Attitude stretch (home-friendly version)

1. Stand tall with one hand resting lightly on a tabletop or chairback.
2. Bend one knee and lift it slightly forward in a soft "attitude" position.
3. Keep your spine neutral as you hinge gently from the crease of your hips.
4. Hold underneath your thigh or rest your ankle lightly on a low ottoman or bench if available for extra support, if needed.
5. Repeat on the other side.

If lifting your leg is challenging, keep it lower; attitude stretches work at any height.

Fold-over running/sassy walk

1. Stand with your feet together.
2. Fold from the crease of your hips, keeping your spine long and neutral.
3. Bend your right knee slightly while lifting your heel, activating the opposite glute.
4. Hold the stretch, then switch sides.
5. Start slowly, then increase tempo once you feel warmed up.

Keep your weight evenly distributed between both feet. Don't drift into the toes.

Hamstring stretch (no-barre version)

1. Stand with your feet together, with one hand lightly touching a countertop or chairback for balance.

2. Step one leg back into a small lunge.

3. Fold forward from your hip crease, keeping your spine long.

4. Flex the toes of your front foot to intensify the hamstring stretch.

5. Repeat on the other side.

If your hamstrings are tight, place your front foot on a low block or thick book for a gentler angle.

Do's and don'ts

» Do hold each stretch for at least two counts of 8.

» Do deepen the stretch gradually on your exhale.

» Don't force your flexibility; let your muscles lengthen naturally.

» Don't round or collapse through your upper back unless the stretch specifically calls for it.

Variations

» Modify by lowering your lifted leg or reducing your fold depth if your balance or flexibility feels limited.

» Progress by increasing your range of motion, adding arm reach or spinal extension when stable, or holding each stretch longer.

» For the pretzel and hamstring stretches, try placing one hand behind your back to open your chest once your balance improves.

Abs and Torso Stretch Series

This floor-based stretch series helps lengthen your abdominals and torso to reduce soreness, improve mobility, and support strong, efficient core work. You'll need a small Pilates ball for one of the stretches. Use this series after your core section or at the end of class to release your torso, calm your nervous system, and restore mobility along your spine and abdominals.

Getting set

Lie on your mat in the center of the floor. Stay relaxed through your shoulders and use your breath to ease deeper into each position.

The movement

Work through the following four stretches, holding each for 16 to 32 counts. This series moves through gentle, supportive positions that help you release your core and torso safely.

Prone stretch

1. Lie on your stomach with your legs extended behind you.

2. Bend your elbows and place your hands slightly wider than your shoulders.

3. Press your hands into the floor as you gently lift your chest.

4. Lengthen through your spine to find a comfortable back extension.

5. Lower and repeat smoothly.

Think of reaching your sternum forward rather than "cranking" upward. This keeps the extension long and safe.

TIP

Ball under lumbar stretch

1. Begin in a bridge position on your back with your knees bent and your arms by your sides.

2. Lift your tailbone just enough to slide a small ball (or a rolled towel or foam roller) under your lumbar spine.

3. Let your pelvis rest on the ball.

4. Choose your leg position: knees bent, legs extended, or knees drawn into your chest.

5. Breathe deeply to release your lower back and hip flexors.

If your lower back feels tense, keep your knees bent, as this is the gentlest on the spine.

TIP

Mermaid stretch

1. Sit with both knees bent to your left side, placing your left hand on your ankles for support.

2. Reach your right arm up toward the ceiling and lengthen up and over to the left (Figure 11-5).

3. Place your right hand on the floor to the right.

4. Sweep your left arm up and over to the right, engaging your oblique muscles to return to center (Figure 11-6).

5. Repeat, then switch sides.

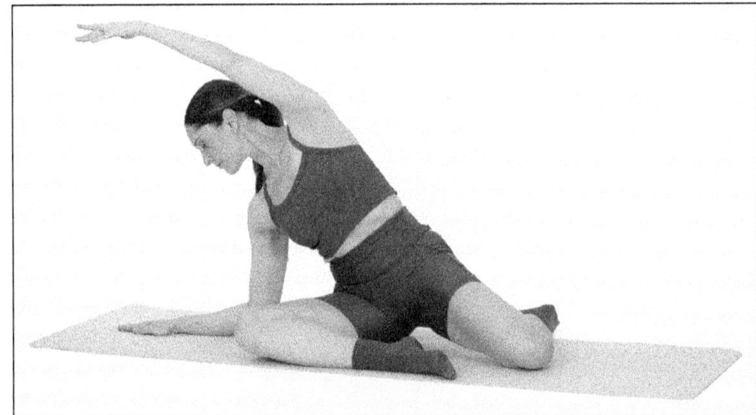

FIGURE 11-5: Reach your right arm up toward the ceiling and lengthen up and over to the left.

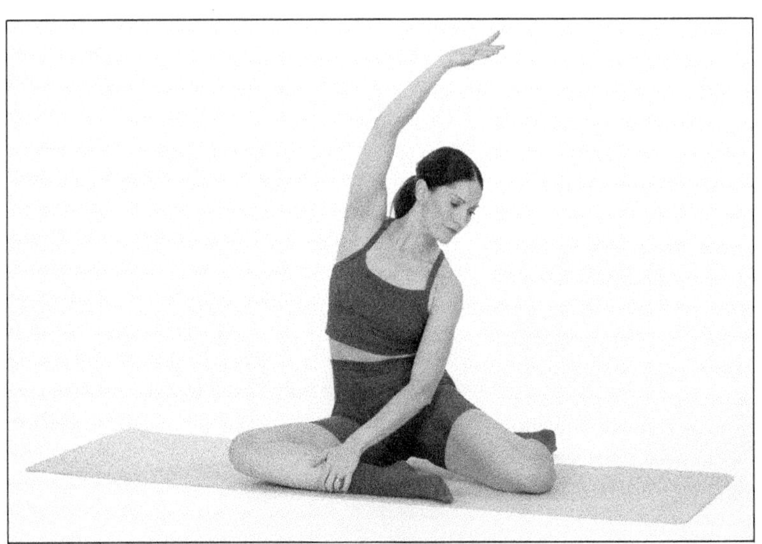

FIGURE 11-6: Sweep your left arm up and over to the right.

Tabletop twist

1. Lie on your back with your knees bent, toes on the floor, and your arms out in a T-position.

2. Gently rotate your lower body to the right as you turn your head to the left (Figure 11-7).

3. Keep both shoulders pressing into the floor.

4. Return to center and switch directions.

5. Repeat smoothly.

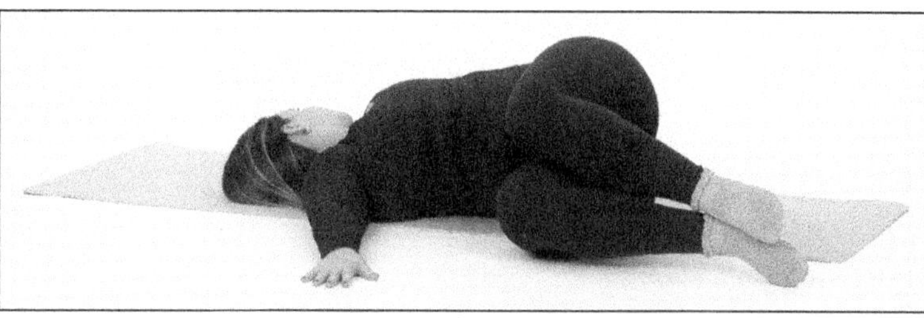

TIP

Move slowly. The slower the twist, the more your spine can relax into rotation.

Do's and don'ts

» Do use your exhale to deepen each stretch gently.

» Do keep your shoulders relaxed and grounded.

» Don't force rotation or extension; let your breath guide your range of motion.

Variations

» Modify by reducing your range of motion or choosing the gentler version of each stretch.

» Progress by lengthening your reach, increasing rotation or extension, or holding each stretch longer.

» For the ball under lumbar stretch, try extending one leg at a time to explore a deeper release.

Full-Body Ballet Stretches

This series of ballet-inspired stretches helps lengthen your glutes, hamstrings, calves, and inner thighs to improve flexibility, prevent injury, and support efficient movement. You can perform all stretches using a chair, countertop, or low table — no barre required.

Use the full-body series at the end of class to release your hips, hamstrings, and inner thighs when they're warm and most responsive to stretching.

Getting set

Stand an arm's distance from a countertop, sturdy chairback, or table. Keep your spine long and your hips square as you prepare to move into each stretch.

The movement

Work through the following four stretches, holding each for 16 to 32 counts. This series moves through simple positions that help your entire lower body release safely and completely.

Parallel leg stretch (flat/round back)

1. Place the arch of one foot on a chair seat or low table in line with your hip.

2. Stand tall with your arms reaching overhead.

3. Hinge forward from the crease of your hips while keeping a long neutral spine.

4. Hold and breathe into the stretch.

5. If your hamstrings feel tight, bring your hands to the chair, table, or your shin.

6. Keep your torso square and avoid rotating your hips.

Think of lengthening your spine forward rather than rounding downward. This keeps the stretch in your hamstrings, not your back.

External rotation side stretch

1. Stand sideways to your support surface (chairback, table, or counter).

2. Externally rotate both legs so that your toes turn slightly outward.

3. Hold your inside hand lightly on the support.

4. Lift your outside arm up and over toward the support surface, lengthening through your side body.

5. Keep both hips rooted and avoid leaning backward.

TIP

Imagine creating space between your ribs as you reach, as this deepens the side bend beautifully.

Thigh and hip stretch (back to support)

1. Stand with your back toward a chair or low table.

2. Place the top of one foot on the chair seat or surface behind you (you can fold a towel under the ankle for comfort).

3. Bring your hands to your hips or lightly touch a countertop for balance.

4. Bend your supporting leg as you press your hips forward to stretch your hip flexor.

5. Keep your spine tall and your pelvis square.

6. Repeat on the other side.

TIP

If placing your foot up feels too intense, keep both feet on the floor and try a long lunge instead.

Penché stretch

1. Stand facing a countertop or sturdy chairback and place your hands lightly on it for balance.

2. Lean forward into a long hinge, keeping your spine neutral.

3. Lift one leg behind you to your comfortable height.

4. Maintain square hips as you tilt forward slightly more to deepen the stretch.

5. Repeat on the other side.

TIP

Lift your back leg only as high as you can without opening your hip. Square alignment matters more than height.

Do's and don'ts

» Do use your exhale to help you ease deeper into each stretch.

» Do keep your hips square and your spine long.

>> Don't force your body into a position that feels sharp or unstable.

>> Don't lock your knees; keep a soft micro-bend if needed.

Variations

>> Modify by lowering the height of your leg (use a lower chair or block) or reducing your fold depth.

>> Progress by increasing your range of motion, lifting your leg slightly higher, or deepening your hinge as flexibility improves.

>> For a gentler option, place your foot on a yoga block instead of a chair.

Floor Stretches

This delicious floor stretch series helps lengthen your glutes, hamstrings, inner thighs, lower back, and calves. These stretches are excellent for improving flexibility, preventing soreness, and resetting your posture after intense lower- or upper-body work.

Use this complete floor series to cool down your legs and lower back at the end of class. These stretches are most effective when your muscles are warm and ready to lengthen.

REMEMBER

Getting set

Sit comfortably on your mat. Lengthen your spine, relax your shoulders, and keep your legs active and aligned as you move through the series. A yoga strap is useful for one of the stretches, but it isn't required.

The movement

Work through the following four stretches, holding each for 16 to 32 counts. This series builds through simple, grounded positions that help you release your entire lower body safely.

Second-position stretch (point/flex)

1. Open your legs wide into a seated second position (Figure 11-8).

2. Reach your left hand up and over toward your right foot.

3. Hold the stretch while flexing both feet to deepen sensation through your calves and inner thighs.

4. Return to center with control.

5. Repeat to the left side.

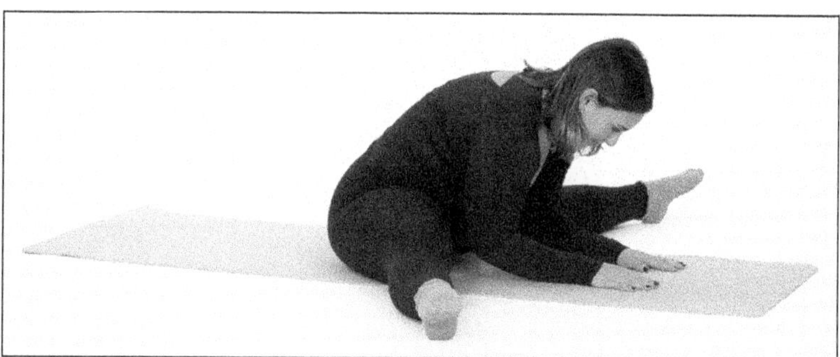

FIGURE 11-8: Start in a seated second position.

Keep both sit bones grounded as you reach, as it keeps the stretch balanced and prevents twisting.

TIP

Single-leg stretch in second position

1. Bend your right knee inward and extend your left leg out to the side in second position.

2. Reach your right arm up and over toward your extended left leg (Figure 11-9).

3. Hold the stretch, breathing deeply.

4. Lift your right arm back up and place it on the floor to your right side.

5. Reach your left arm overhead and gently lift your pelvis to bring your spine into a light extension.

6. Lower down with control and repeat on the other side.

Press gently into your supporting hand during the extension. It helps keep your chest open without collapsing into your lower back.

TIP

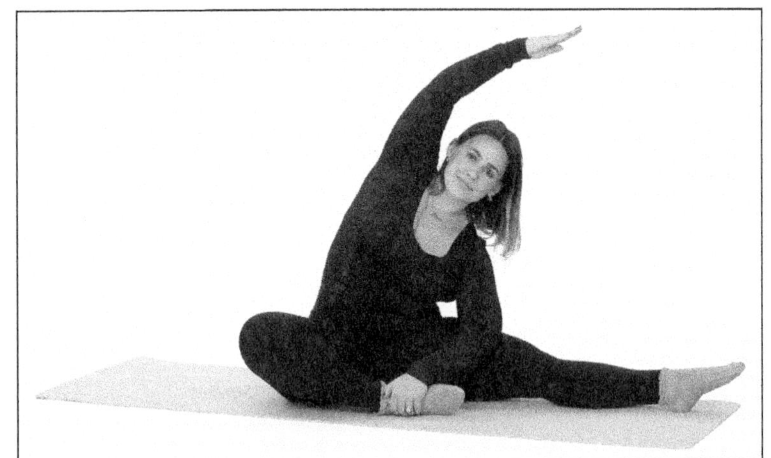

Forward fold with point/flex

1. Extend both legs straight in front of you with your feet parallel.

2. Hinge forward from the crease of your hips to reach toward your feet or shins (Figure 11-10).

3. Alternate flexing and pointing your toes to change the stretch through your calves and hamstrings.

4. Stay long through your spine and avoid rounding excessively.

5. Slowly articulate your spine to return to a tall, seated position.

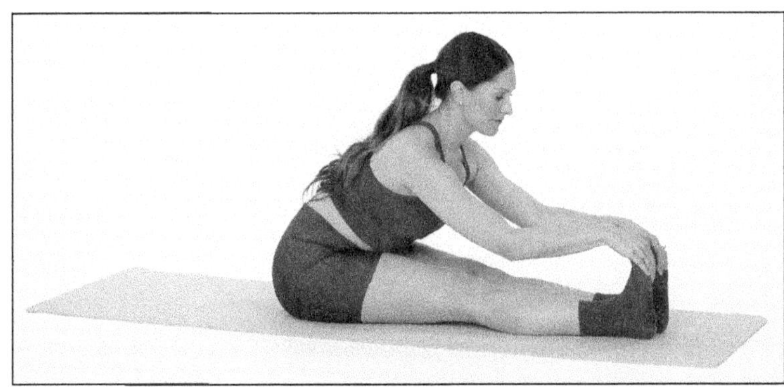

Yoga strap series (parallel, external rotation, internal rotation)

1. Lie on your back with both legs extended.

2. Loop a yoga strap around the arch of one foot.

   You can use a long, folded towel instead of a yoga strap.

3. Lift your leg toward the ceiling in parallel alignment, holding the stretch.

4. Open your leg outward into external rotation while keeping your opposite hip grounded.

5. Bring the leg across your body into internal rotation for a gentle IT-band and outer-hip stretch.

6. Repeat on the other leg.

Move your leg only as far as you can keep your pelvis stable. Less is more if it helps maintain alignment!

Do's and don'ts

>> Do use your exhale to deepen each stretch gradually.

>> Do keep both sit bones anchored whenever possible.

>> Don't force your legs into a range that creates strain in your knees or lower back.

Variations

>> Modify by decreasing your range of motion or softening your knees if your hamstrings feel tight.

>> Progress by widening your second position, reaching farther, or holding each stretch longer.

>> In the strap series, try circling your lifted leg slowly to mobilize your hip joint further.

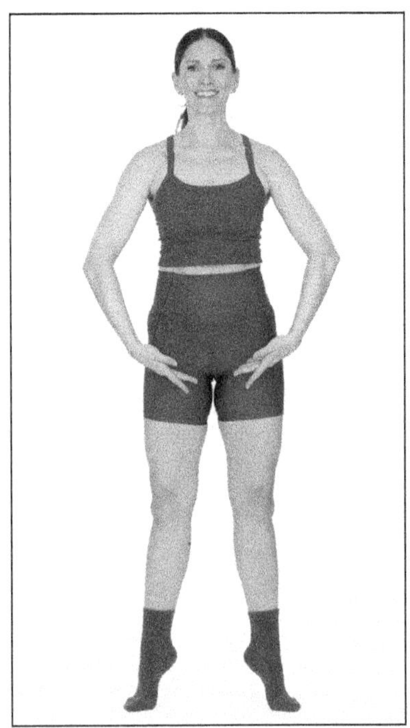

Balance Ending

This simple but powerful balance sequence strengthens your stability, posture, and mind-body awareness. It's a grounding way to finish class and incorporate all the techniques you have learned into one final moment of control.

Getting set

Stand in the center of the floor with your feet in a parallel stance or in first position. Let your arms rest by your sides or hold in a low fifth position, as shown in Figure 11-11, and prepare to move with slow, steady control.

The movement

Hold each stage of this sequence for 15 to 30 counts. This closing series unfolds through simple, centered steps that help you finish class with balance and intention.

1. **Start with a high relevé balance.**

   a. Lift both heels to rise into a high relevé.

   b. Engage your inner thighs and draw your core upward.

   c. Lift both arms smoothly into high fifth position overhead.

   d. Hold your balance with steady breath and lifted posture.

Instantly improve your balance by imagining a string lifting the crown of your head.

2. **Move into head turns.**

   a. Still holding your relevé (or parallel balance), gently turn your head to the left for one count.

   b. Gently turn to the right for one count.

   c. Return your gaze to the center without wobbling through your torso.

Gently move your head, not your shoulders. The challenge is to keep the rest of your body perfectly still.

3. **Finish with a controlled lower and reset.**

   a. Lower your heels carefully with control.

   b. Bring your arms down to your sides.

   c. Roll your shoulders back four times to release tension and reset your posture.

This final balance is designed to center your energy, integrate your technique, and leave you feeling tall, strong, and connected. Take a deep breath as you complete your practice.

Do's and don'ts

» Do focus on core control, balance, and alignment.

» Do lift through your spine without locking your knees.

» Don't grip your toes or let your weight fall backward.

» Don't rush the lowering. Control is the final cue of the workout.

Variations

>> Keep your heels on the floor if balancing on relevé feels unstable.

>> Progress by practicing the sequence in first position, fifth position, or parallel to challenge different stabilizers.

>> Try adding a soft arm port de bras before returning to high fifth position once you're comfortable with the balance.

3 Workouts That (Really) Work

Work through three 50-minute full-body workouts that provide variety while building strength, balance, and confidence.

Work through a shorter 30-minute workout on busy days that still lifts your heart rate and strengthens your whole body.

Discover how 15-minute express workouts offer a quick hit of strength that leaves you feeling lifted, energized, and ready to take on the world.

Explore how you can add "movement snacks" to your day to wake up your muscles and reset your posture, no matter where you are or what you are doing.

Chapter **12**

Full-Body Workouts

Welcome to one of my favorite parts of this book. These full-body workouts come straight from my studio method and have been tried and loved by thousands of clients looking to feel strong, balanced, and energized. Whether you choose a 50-minute session for the full experience (choosing between Workout A, B, or C) or a 30-minute option for busy days, each workout delivers targeted movement that makes a real difference.

REMEMBER

The moves may be small, but that's the secret. Precise, controlled motion helps you activate muscles deeply and safely, building strength and improving posture and mobility over time. With consistency, these short sequences create big changes.

Before you begin each workout, make sure your space is clear and safe, and listen to your body as you move. No matter which workout you choose today, you are about to feel more connected, confident, and capable. Are you ready to go?

Full-Body 50-Minute Workout A

This is one of my signature full-body workouts from my studio method — my go-to sequences for building strength, balance, and confidence. The movements may look small, but they create big results when you stay focused and consistent. Set up your space so that you can move freely, take a breath to center yourself, and let's get started.

What you need

Here is what I recommend having nearby for this workout:

>> A mat

>> Optional light hand weights

>> Small Pilates ball

>> Resistance band

>> A chair, countertop, or yoga stick for balance

How to do it

I designed this sequence so that each section builds on the last. Move through it in order, stay mindful of your form, and take breaks as needed.

Warm-up

5 minutes

I like to think of the warm-up as your invitation into the workout. These moves wake up your muscles gently while preparing your joints for the more targeted work ahead.

>> Knee-lift series: 4 sets, 8 counts each

>> Plié tendu: 8 to 16 counts

>> Side reach: 2 slow repetitions plus 8 to 16 at tempo

Upper-body series

10 to 12 minutes

This upper-body section always surprises people. The movements look tiny, but the burn arrives quickly and safely because the moves are so targeted.

>> Biceps curls front: 8 to 16 repetitions

>> 90-degree lifts: 8 to 16 repetitions

>> Open and close series: 8 to 16 repetitions

- >> Puppet: 8 to 16 repetitions

- >> Biceps curls side: 8 to 16 repetitions

- >> Arm circles side: 8 to 16 repetitions

- >> Swimming series: 2 slow repetitions plus 8 to 16 at tempo

- >> Curtsy triceps or triceps lunges: 2 slow plus 8 to 16 at tempo

Next, you'll transition to the mat, where you'll shift into deeper upper-body and core strength. It is a quick section, but it is powerful and incredibly effective.

- >> Triceps lunges: 16 to 32 repetitions

- >> Push-ups center floor: 16 to 32 repetitions

- >> Plank (any variation): 60 seconds

TIP

Upper-body stretches: It's important to stretch the upper body here to release tension and prepare for the lower-body work ahead. Try a set of elbow draw-downs (Figure 12-1), then flow into a chest expansion (Figure 12-2), arm cross-overs (Figure 12-3), and a standing side bend connecting with one wrist after the other (Figure 12-4).

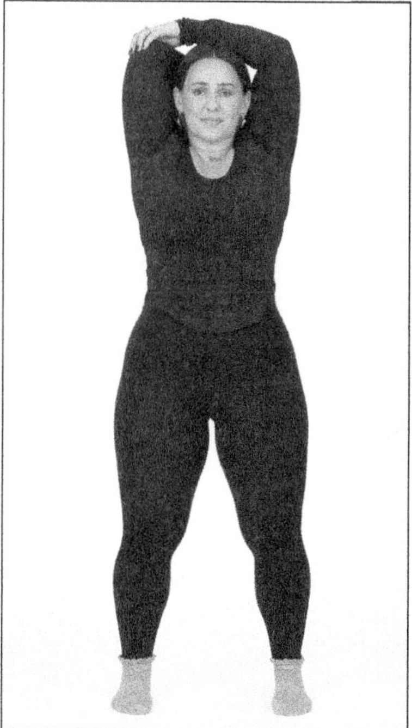

FIGURE 12-1: Elbow draw-downs.

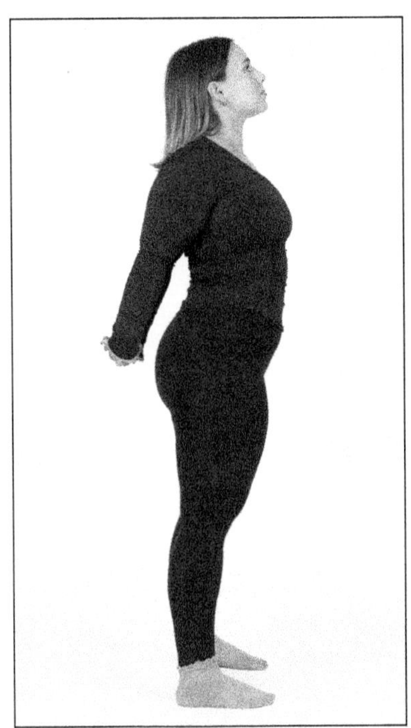

FIGURE 12-2:
Chest expansion.

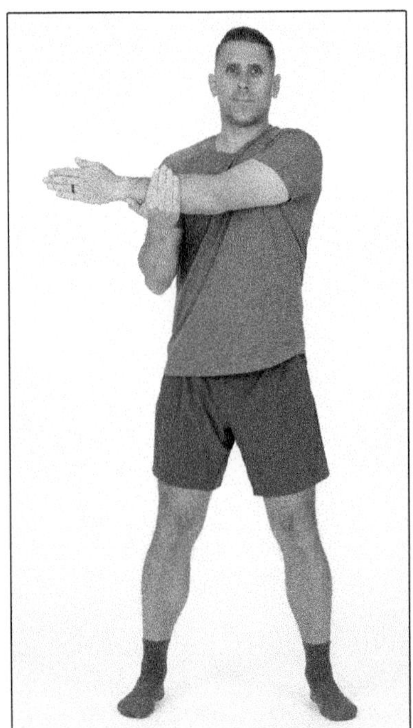

FIGURE 12-3:
Arm cross-overs.

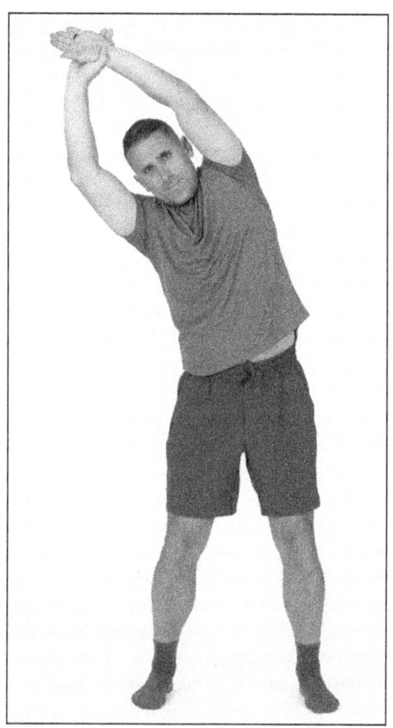

Barre series

25 minutes

This is where the classic studio magic happens. These small, precise movements are what give Barre its reputation. When you focus on form, the results come quickly.

Thigh work

>> First-position relevé and pliés on relevé: 16 to 32 repetitions

>> Second-position cardio: 2 to 3 variations, 8 to 16 repetitions each

>> Parallel pliés with ball pulse: 16 to 32 repetitions

>> Hip circles with ball: 16 to 32 repetitions

TIP

Thigh stretches: Add a hip flexor stretch here (Figure 12-5) to help your muscles reset before you continue.

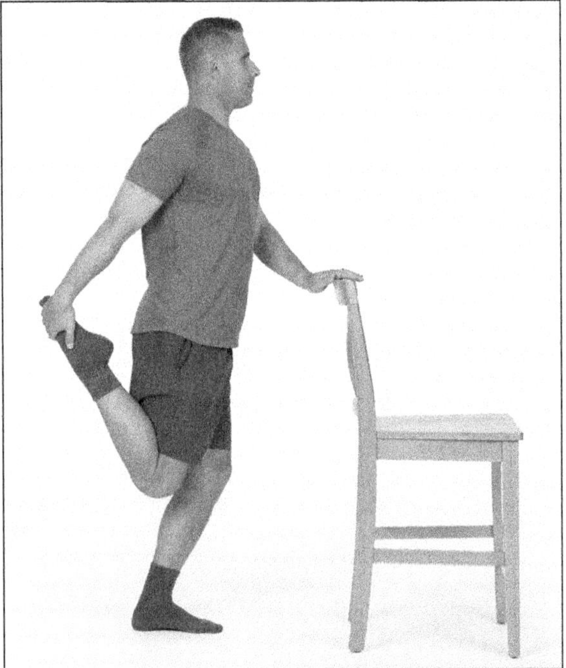

FIGURE 12-5:
Hip flexor stretch.

Resistance-band series

This short series uses a resistance band to add challenge without impact. The band gives you feedback on alignment while lighting up your glutes, hips, and outer thighs in that very Barre way.

>> Choose 2 to 3 resistance-band exercises (such as open and close, leg circles, or side presses), performing 8 to 16 repetitions of each before moving on.

>> Add walks and cardio: Include 2 to 3 variations of banded side walks or quick pulses, doing 8 to 16 repetitions each to raise the heart rate and deepen the burn. Think strong, controlled, and slightly spicy.

Fold-over series

Fold-over work is one of my studio favorites because it's safe, targeted, and incredibly effective for the entire back line of the body, especially the hamstrings, glutes, and lower back.

You'll see many of these fold-over variations throughout the workouts in this book. Here, you're simply choosing a few favorites and linking them together.

>> Choose 2 to 3 fold-over exercises, performing 8 to 16 repetitions of each before moving on.

>> Add variations of your choice, such as small pulses, heel lifts, single-leg bends, or a gentle twist, for 8 to 16 repetitions per set.

Keep the spine long, the movement controlled, and the focus inward. These are small moves with big payoff, and yes, they tend to sneak up on you.

Seat stretches: This is your moment to release the seat muscles after all that focused work.

Core series

10 minutes

I design my core section to build strength from the inside out. Every movement here supports your posture and your overall stability.

>> C-curve hold: 16 to 32 seconds

>> Supine lifts: 8 to 16 repetitions per set

>> Scissor crisscross: 16 repetitions

Abdominal stretches: The tabletop stretch (Figure 12-6) and the second-position floor stretch (Figure 12-7) help reset the hip flexors and abdominal muscles after deep core work.

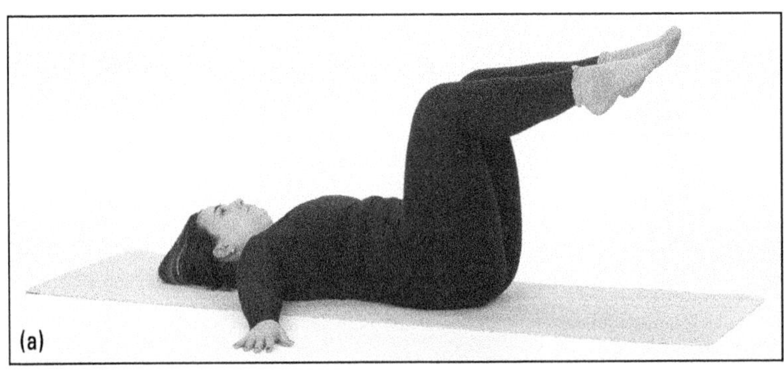

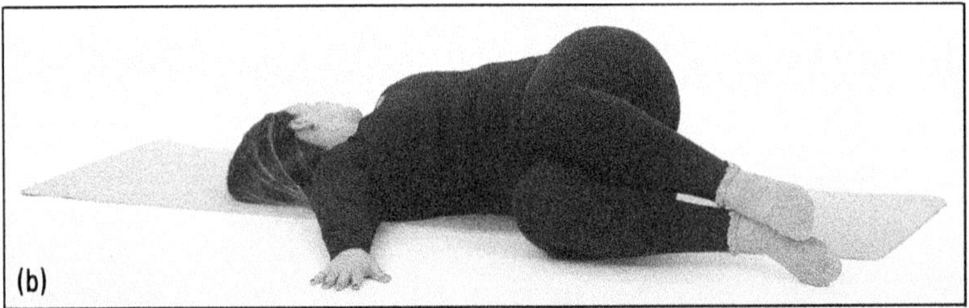

FIGURE 12-6: Tabletop twist stretch starting position (a) and twist (b).

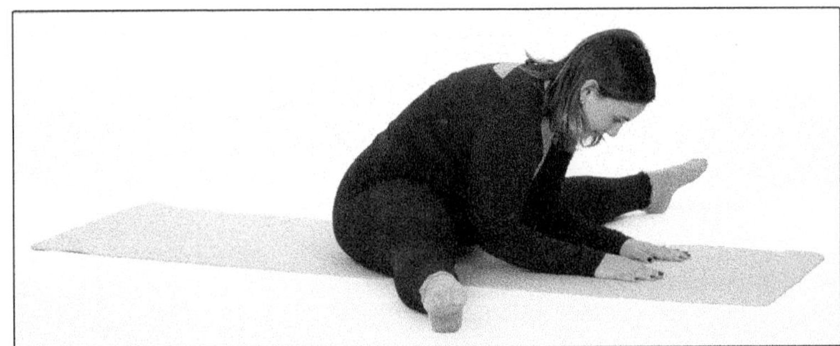

FIGURE 12-7: Second-position floor stretch.

Lower-body floor series

2 to 4 minutes

Choose the option that feels best for your body today. Both options activate and strengthen the glutes safely.

>> Side-seat series: 8 to 16 repetitions per set

or

>> Bottoms up: 8 to 16 repetitions per set

Stretches and balance ending

3 to 5 minutes

I always finish class with stretching and a balance ending so that your body has time to reset and absorb the work you've just done. This is where everything settles. Your muscles lengthen, your nervous system calms down, and you leave feeling taller, steadier, and quietly proud of yourself.

Choose 2 to 4 stretches, holding each for slow, steady breaths:

>> Thigh and hip stretch to release the front of the legs after pliés and lunges

>> Hamstring fold-over to lengthen the back of the body

>> Seat or figure-four stretch to ease the hips and glutes

>> Upper-body stretch, such as chest expansion, triceps stretch, or side reach

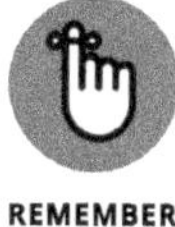

REMEMBER

Move slowly here. This is not about pushing flexibility; it's about recovery and integration.

Finish with a balance ending, which is a short standing balance sequence that brings everything together. Typically, this includes:

>> Standing tall in parallel or first position

>> Rising to a controlled relevé

>> Holding balance while engaging the core and inner thighs

>> Adding a simple arm position or a gentle head turn

>> Lowering with control and rolling the shoulders out

The balance ending is both physical and mental. It reinforces posture, focus, and stability, and it gives your body a clear signal that the workout is complete. End class with these stretches and the balance ending so that you leave feeling tall, centered, and confident. Figure 12-8 and Figure 12-9 show two variations of the balance ending.

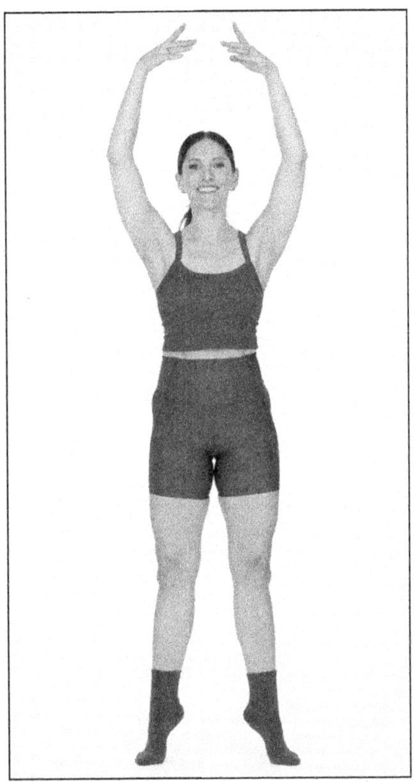

Full-Body 50-Minute Workout B

For variety, this full-body workout feels steady, strong, and incredibly satisfying. The movements follow a smooth progression that warms your body, challenges your strength, and finishes with the slow burn Barre is known for. Even though the moves may look simple, they are precise and intentional, and you will absolutely feel them working. Clear your space, take a breath, and let's get moving.

What you need

Here is what I like to keep close for this workout:

>> A mat

>> Optional light hand weights

>> A chair, countertop, or yoga stick for balance

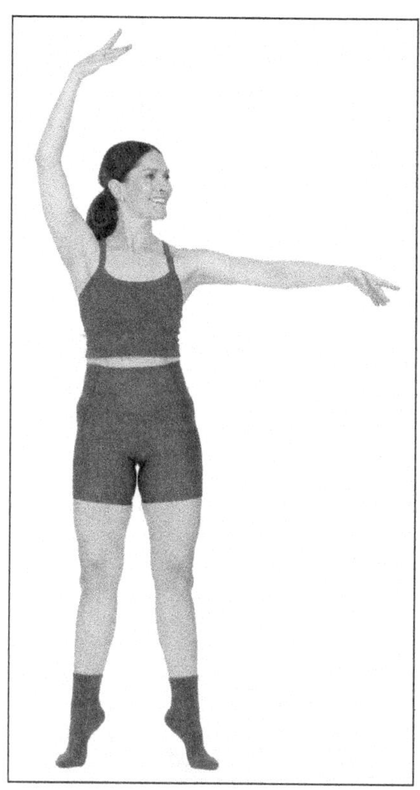

How to do it

I designed this workout to flow naturally from warm-up to strength work to stretching. Move section by section, stay aware of your posture, and enjoy the rhythm of the routine.

Warm-up

5 minutes

I use this warm-up to wake up the body gently while setting the tone for the rest of the class. Everything is simple and steady so that you can prepare your muscles for the more focused work ahead.

>> Knee lifts: 8 repetitions each set, up to 4 sets

>> First-position lunge back: 8 to 16 repetitions per set

>> Curtsy pliés: 8 to 16 repetitions per set

Upper-body series

10 to 12 minutes

This upper-body sequence builds strength through small, controlled movements. I love this series because it tones without strain and helps improve posture from the inside out.

>> Arm circles: 16 repetitions in each direction

>> Bicep curls: 8 to 16 repetitions

>> 90-degree lifts: 8 to 16 repetitions

>> Rowing: 8 to 16 repetitions

>> Hug and carriage: 8 repetitions, alternating sides

>> Waltzing: 8 to 16 repetitions

>> Triceps lunges: 8 to 16 repetitions, up to 2 sets

Next, I bring you down to the mat to strengthen your upper body and core in a way that feels grounded and supported.

>> Triceps lunges: 8 to 16 repetitions, up to 2 sets

>> Push-ups center floor: 16 to 32 repetitions

Upper-body stretches: Take a moment to stretch here so that your upper body feels loose, open, and ready for the lower-body work that comes next. Refer to Figures 12-1, 12-2, 12-3, and 12-4 in Workout A for the stretches to do.

Barre series

25 minutes

This is the heart of the workout. These movements are classic, controlled, and incredibly effective for shaping your thighs, glutes, and hips. Even the smallest range will leave you feeling strong and powerful.

Thigh work

I begin with foundational thigh exercises that build heat quickly and safely.

>> First-position pliés: 8 to 16 repetitions, up to 2 sets

>> Passé press: 8 to 16 repetitions, up to 2 sets

>> Second-position pliés: 8 to 16 repetitions, up to 2 sets

>> Back to barre battements: 8 to 16 repetitions

>> Side lifts: 16 to 32 counts

>> Second-position cardio: 16 repetitions, 1 or 2 variations

Thigh stretches: This quick stretch helps release tension so that you can move with better range and control. (See Figure 12-5 for the hip flexor stretch.)

Fold-over series

This section strengthens the back of your body with controlled, precise movements that create a deep, supportive burn.

>> Choose two to three fold-over variations: 8 to 16 repetitions per set, up to 2 sets

Suggested fold-over variations:

>> Parallel fold-over with soft knees, hinging from the hips and maintaining a long spine (Figure 12-10)

>> Running fold-over by gently bending one knee while lifting the opposite heel, then switching sides

>> Wide second position fold-over to target inner thighs and hamstrings (Figure 12-11)

>> Knee to elbow fold-over to add light core engagement and coordination

>> Flat back to round back fold-over to mobilize the spine while strengthening the posterior chain

Seat stretches: This is your moment to open the hips and glutes after all the focused lower-body work.

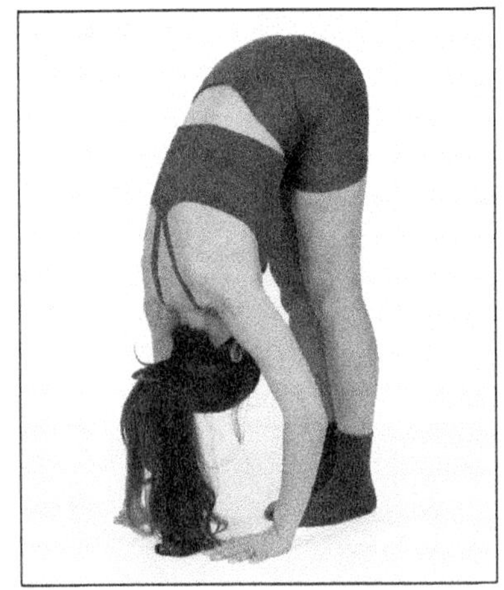

FIGURE 12-10: A standing fold-over with soft knees, palms on the floor.

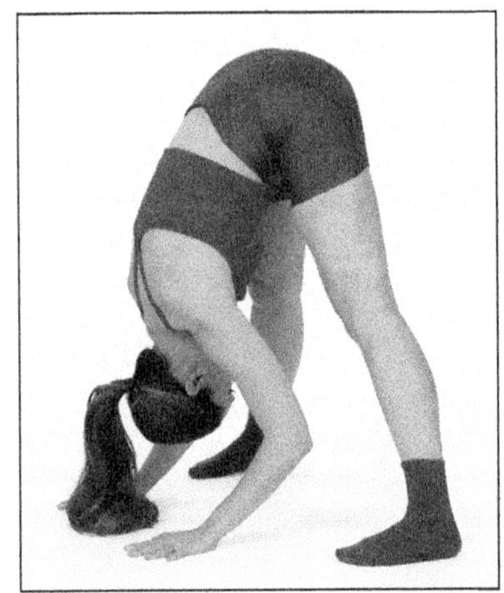

FIGURE 12-11: A wide second-position fold-over to target inner thighs and hamstrings.

Core series

10 minutes

This core flow builds deep abdominal strength and improves your stability. Every exercise supports your posture and helps you move with more confidence.

>> C-curve hold: 8 to 16 counts

>> C-curve abs: 8 to 16 repetitions per set

» Passé abs: 8 repetitions per set

» Scissor crisscross: 16 repetitions

» Plank (any variation): 60 seconds

Abdominal stretches: Be sure to stretch the core here to keep your spine long and your hip flexors open after all the abdominal work. Refer to Figures 12-6 and 12-7 in Workout A for the tabletop twist stretch and the second-position floor stretch.

Lower-body floor series

2 to 4 minutes

Here is one more chance to strengthen the lower body safely while staying grounded.

» Bottoms up: 8 to 16 repetitions per set

Stretches and balance ending

3 to 5 minutes

Finish with the full-body stretches to lengthen the muscles you have worked, and the final balance described in Workout A to help you feel centered and lifted. This is your moment to slow down and acknowledge the strength you built today.

Full-Body 50-Minute Workout C

This workout is one of my go-to routines when I want to feel energized and athletic from head to toe. The pace is a little more dynamic, and you will move through a variety of pliés, lunges, lifts, and core work that keep your muscles guessing. Even though so many of the movements are small, they pack a powerful punch when you stay focused. Make sure your space is clear, your footing feels secure, and you are ready to move with intention.

What you need

Here is what I recommend keeping nearby for this workout:

» A mat

» Optional light hand weights

» A chair, countertop, or yoga stick for balance

How to do it

I designed this routine to build intensity gradually. Move through each section in order and stay connected to your form so that the work stays safe and effective.

Warm-up

5 minutes

This warm-up blends familiar Barre movements with gentle mobility work to prepare your body for more focused exercises. Take your time and allow the heat to build naturally.

» Plié tendu: 8 repetitions each set, up to 4 sets

» Side reach: 8 to 16 repetitions per set

» Curtsy pliés: 8 repetitions per set

Upper-body series

10 to 12 minutes

This upper-body block has a playful feel. The arm positions shift often, which keeps your shoulders awake and helps you build strength through a full range of motion.

» Bicep curls: 8 to 16 repetitions

» Arm circles: 8 to 16 repetitions

» Hug and carriage: 8 repetitions, alternating sides

>> Swimming series: 8 repetitions

>> Triceps lunges: 8 to 16 repetitions, up to 2 sets

Next, you'll transition to the mat where you'll begin to engage your upper body and core from a grounded position.

>> Triceps lunges: 8 to 16 repetitions, up to 2 sets

>> Push-ups center floor: 16 to 32 repetitions

Upper-body stretches: Pause here and stretch to keep your posture tall and your shoulders relaxed before moving into the Barre section. Refer to Figures 12-1, 12-2, 12-3, and 12-4 in Workout A for the stretches to do.

Barre series

25 minutes

This section blends strength, balance, and endurance. The movements are simple but deeply effective when you hold your alignment steady.

Thigh work

These exercises warm the legs quickly while training stability through your hips and core.

>> Parallel pliés: 8 repetitions, up to 2 sets

>> Second-position cardio: 2 sets of 8 repetitions per series

>> Hip circles: 8 to 16 repetitions per set, up to 2 sets

>> Back to barre battements: 8 to 16 repetitions, up to 2 sets

Thigh stretches: Take a moment for a quick release to stay loose and maintain good form as you continue. (See Figure 12-5 for the hip flexor stretch.)

Glute and hip work

These movements target the glutes and outer hips with slow, controlled strength work.

>> Hamstring series: 8 repetitions, up to 2 sets

>> Fourth-position pliés: 8 to 16 repetitions, up to 2 sets

>> Fold-over series: 8 repetitions per set, up to 2 sets

Seat stretches: Let your hips open here. This stretch is especially helpful after the side lifts and fold-over work.

Core series

10 minutes

This core flow strengthens your deep abdominals and improves your posture. The movements may look simple, but when you focus on your breath and alignment, they become incredibly effective.

>> C-curve hold: 8 to 16 counts

>> Passé abs: 8 to 16 repetitions each side

>> Supine lifts: 8 to 16 repetitions each side

>> Plank (any variation): 60 seconds

Abdominal stretches: These stretches help open the front of your body and balance the deep core work you just completed. Refer to Figures 12-6 and 12-7 in Workout A for the tabletop twist stretch and the second-position floor stretch.

Lower-body floor series

2 to 4 minutes

This is your final lower-body challenge.

>> Pretzels: 8 to 16 repetitions per set

Stretches and balance ending

3 to 5 minutes

Finish by stretching your full body to release the muscles you have worked. Then take a final balance to steady your mind and leave the workout feeling aligned and confident. Refer to Workout A for the full-body stretches and balance ending.

Full-Body 30-Minute Workout

There are days when a full workout just is not in the cards, and that is exactly why I love this shorter version. In only 30 minutes, you can lift your heart rate, strengthen your whole body, and finish feeling refreshed and accomplished. Even though this session is shorter, the targeted movements still give you everything you need. Clear your space, take a deep breath, and let's get moving.

What you need

Here is what I like to keep nearby for this quick session:

>> A mat

>> Optional light hand weights

>> A chair, countertop, or yoga stick for balance

How to do it

This workout moves at a steady, efficient pace. Follow each section in order and focus on clean form so you get the most out of every minute.

Warm up

5 minutes

This warm-up quickly wakes up your whole body so that you can dive straight into the express format without feeling rushed.

>> Plié tendu with high-V arms and battement: 8 to 16 repetitions

>> Curtsy pliés: 2 slow, then 8 repetitions at tempo

>> Side-reach series: 2 side tendus, 2 side passés, and 1 side battement

Add light weights if you want more challenge.

Upper-body series

10 minutes

In this 30-minute workout, I like to blend upper-body and lower-body movements to keep your heart rate up. Simple leg positions or gentle lunges help create a full-body challenge.

>> Bicep curls or 90-degree lifts: 8 to 16 repetitions (Optional: Add a high-low lower-body pattern or small jumps)

>> Open and close from first to second position: 8 to 16 repetitions; hold in second position at the end

>> Swimming series: 8 to 16 repetitions

>> Curtsy triceps: 8 to 16 repetitions

Deepen your pliés or lift your front heel to advance the work.

Barre series

15 to 18 minutes

This section is packed with efficient movements to work your legs, hips, and glutes. Even small ranges of motion will build heat fast.

>> Second-position pliés: 8 to 16 repetitions (Optional: Open and close to First position or add gentle jumps)

>> Side lift: 8 to 16 repetitions; lift and lower your outer leg to target the side seat and obliques

>> Passé press plus second-position cardio combo: 8 to 16 repetitions; lift, press, and add gentle cardio variations to increase intensity

>> Fold-over series or fold-over lunges: 8 to 16 repetitions

Choose the variation that feels best for your body today.

Core series

3 to 5 minutes

This express core sequence is fast, focused, and incredibly effective.

>> Plank: 30 seconds; add knee-to-chest (8 each side), step-outs (8 each side), or plank jumps (8 repetitions), depending on your level and how you are feeling today

>> Lifts: 8 to 16 repetitions

>> Scissors crisscross: 8 to 16 repetitions

Use a hover under the leg for added core stability.

Stretches and balance ending

2 to 3 minutes

Finish by stretching your whole body to cool down, release tension, and restore mobility. Close with a final balance to reconnect with your posture and center yourself before moving on with your day.

Chapter **13**

Express Workouts

L et's be honest. Most days, life does not hand you a neat, uninterrupted hour to work out. That's exactly when these express workouts come in handy. Each workout in this chapter is short, focused, and super effective. They're built around the idea I come back to again and again: Small, intentional actions add up. These sessions zero in on one area of the body at a time, so you can drop in, get to work, and feel that spicy Barre burn without overthinking or overplanning.

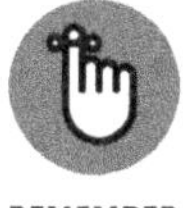

Don't be fooled by the length. These workouts are precise, targeted, and tough in the best possible way. You'll use the same Barre principles you've learned throughout the book, just condensed into a faster format that still builds strength, alignment, and confidence.

REMEMBER

Express Upper-Body Workout

Some days you just need a quick hit of strength, the kind that makes you feel lifted, energized, and ready to take on the world. This upper-body express workout delivers exactly that. These small but mighty movements come straight from my studio, and they sneak up on you fast. By the end, your posture will feel brighter, your arms will feel sculpted, and your confidence will get a boost. Clear your space and let's give your upper body some love.

What you need

Here is what I recommend having nearby for this workout:

>> Light hand weights (optional)

>> A mat

>> A chair or countertop for balance

How to do it

Follow the sequence without rushing. Small movements make a big impact.

Warm-up

1 to 2 minutes

>> Shoulder rolls: 8 forward, 8 back

>> Arm sweeps: 6 to 8 repetitions

>> March with oppositional arms: 30 seconds

Upper-body sculpt

10 minutes

>> Bicep curls: 12 to 16 repetitions

>> 90-degree lifts: 12 repetitions

>> V-press: 12 repetitions

>> Arm circles: 16 to 20 each way

>> Genie arms: 12 repetitions

>> Triceps lunge (Figure 13-1): 16 repetitions each arm

>> Swimming arms: 30 seconds

>> Temperature arms: 12 repetitions

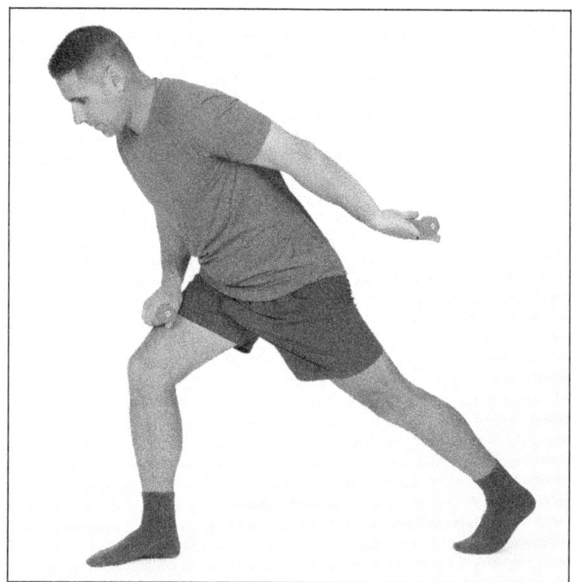

Optional cardio burst

1 minute

>> Overhead reach and pull: 30 seconds

>> Open and close arms: 30 seconds

Balance

30 seconds

>> Rise to toes and reach overhead

Stretch

2 minutes

>> Cross-body stretch

>> Triceps stretch

>> Chest expansion

>> Deep breath overhead

Express Lower-Body Workout

Your legs and glutes are some of the biggest, strongest muscles in your body, which means even a short workout can deliver big results. This express lower-body session wakes up your hips, thighs, and seat with movements that look simple but work deeply. You will build heat quickly, feel stronger with every rep, and stand taller by the end. Grab balance support if you need it, and let's fire up your lower half.

What you need

Here is what I recommend having nearby for this workout:

>> A mat

>> A chair or countertop for balance

How to do it

Stay steady and controlled. Form matters more than speed.

Warm-up

1 to 2 minutes

>> Knee-lift march: 30 seconds

>> Mini squats: 10 repetitions

>> Side-step touch: 30 seconds

Lower-body sculpt

10 minutes

>> Second-position pliés: 12 to 16 repetitions

>> Second-position pulses: 20 repetitions

>> Chair position: 12 repetitions

>> Chair heel lifts: 12 each side

>> Lunge backs: 8 to 10 each side

>> Side leg lifts: 12 to 16 each side

>> Knee to elbow crunch: 30 seconds

>> Fold-over glute lift (Figure 13-2): 12 to 16 repetitions each leg

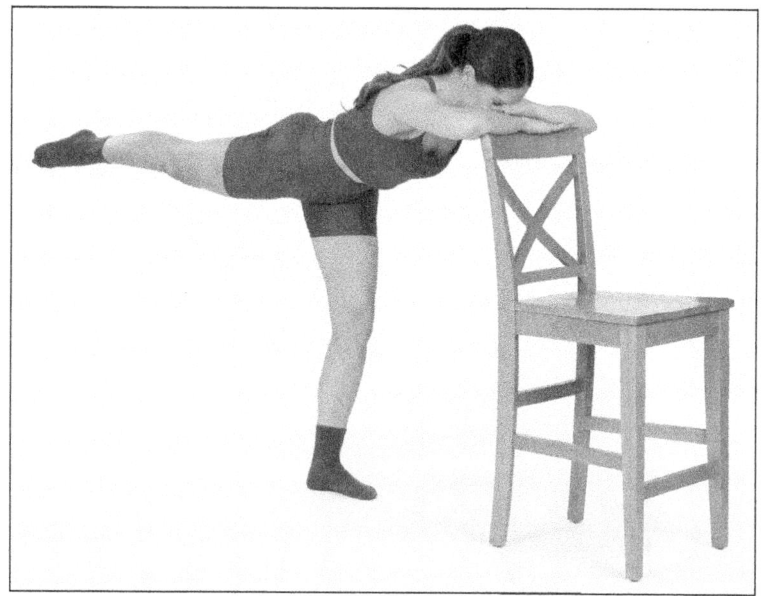

Optional cardio burst

1 minute

>> Second-position squat reach: 30 seconds

>> Alternating reverse lunge: 30 seconds

Balance

30 seconds

>> Passé hold

Stretch

2 minutes

- **»** Quad stretch

- **»** Hamstring stretch

- **»** Figure-four stretch (Figure 13-3)

- **»** Big deep breath

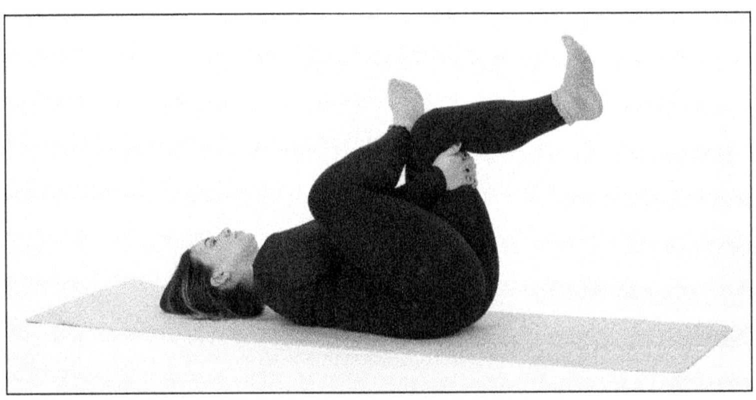

FIGURE 13-3: Lift your legs to the tabletop position, rest one ankle on your knee, and lace your fingers behind that same knee for support. Remember to breathe.

Express Core Workout

A strong core supports everything you do, from standing tall to carrying groceries with ease. This express core workout targets the deep abdominal muscles that stabilize your spine and improve your everyday movement. The exercises are small and focused, classic Barre magic that builds strength quickly without overwhelming your body. You will be surprised how centered and powerful you feel in just 15 minutes.

What you need

Here is what I recommend having nearby for this workout:

- **»** A mat. That's it!

How to do it

Focus on smooth breathing and controlled movement.

Warm-up

1 minute

>> March with core engagement: 30 seconds

>> Standing side bends: 20 seconds

Core series

10 minutes

>> C-curve hold (Figure 13-4): 10 to 15 seconds

>> C-curve pulses: 12 to 16 repetitions

>> Oblique twists: 12 to 16 repetitions

>> Supine marches: 12 repetitions each leg

>> Plank passé (Figure 13-5): 8 to 10 repetitions

>> Scissors: 12 to 16 repetitions

>> Crisscross: 12 to 16 repetitions

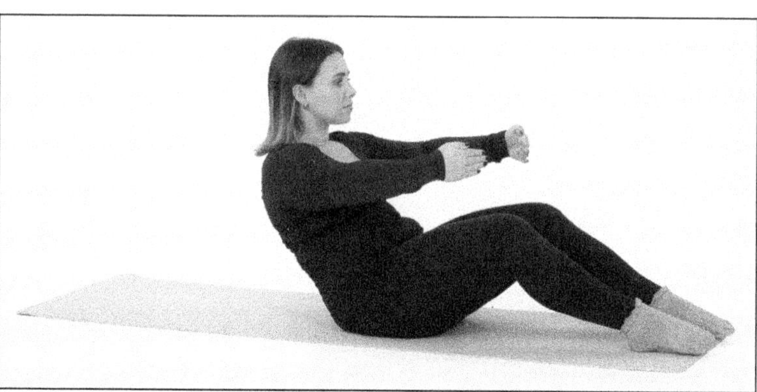

FIGURE 13-4: Hold a C-curve for 10 to 15 seconds.

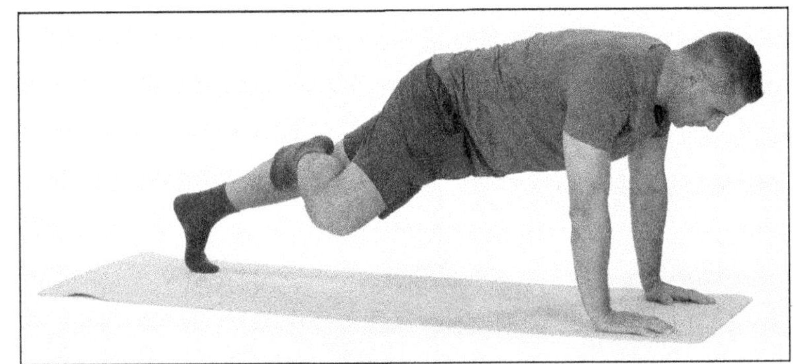

Optional core cardio

1 minute

>> Mountain climbers: 30 seconds

>> Plank walkouts: 30 seconds

Balance

30 seconds

>> Knee-lift balance with arms overhead

Stretch

2 minutes

>> Prone extension (Figure 13-6)

>> Seated side stretch

>> Lying twist

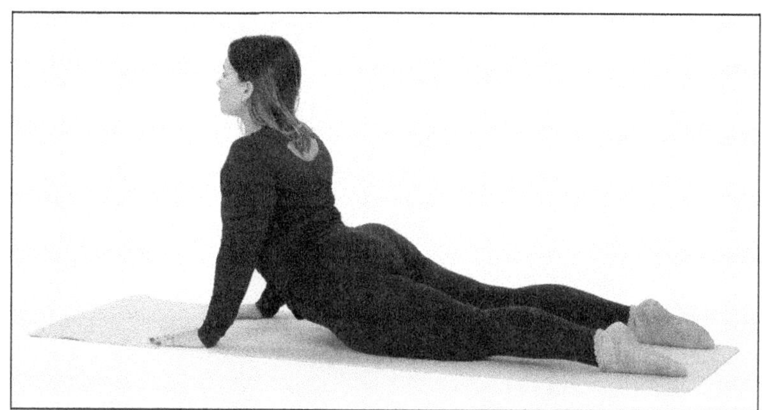

Express Cardio Workout

When you want a quick mood-boost and a burst of energy, this express cardio workout is your go-to. The movements are simple and upbeat, helping you raise your heart rate without complicated choreography. It is designed to make you feel light, refreshed, and empowered in just 15 minutes. Think of it as a reset button for your whole body.

What you need

Here is what I recommend having nearby for this workout:

>> A mat (optional)

How to do it

Stay light on your feet and move with intention.

Warm-up

1 minute

>> March with reach: 30 seconds

>> Step touch with arm sweep: 30 seconds

Cardio series

10 minutes

> » Second-position plié and reach: 30 seconds
>
> » Standing knee pulls: 30 seconds
>
> » Side-to-side lunge reach: 30 seconds
>
> » Curtsy with side lift: 30 seconds
>
> » Jog or march in place: 30 seconds
>
> » Knee to elbow twist: 30 seconds
>
> » Parallel squat and arm swing: 30 seconds

Repeat this cycle once.

Balance

30 seconds

> » Hold second position, arms overhead

Stretch

2 minutes

> » Hamstring stretch
>
> » Quad stretch
>
> » Overhead reach

Express Total-Body Workout

If you want a little bit of everything in one quick session — sculpting, cardio, and balance — this total-body express workout is for you. These movements come straight from my studio method and are loved because they work quickly without taking over your day. By the end, you'll feel strong, lifted, and recharged, ready to move on with renewed energy.

What you need

Here is what I recommend having nearby for this workout:

>> Light weights (optional)

>> A mat

>> A chair or countertop for balance

How to do it

Stay present and enjoy the flow of fast transitions.

Warm-up

1 minute

>> March with arm sweep: 30 seconds

>> Mini pliés: 30 seconds

Total-body sculpt

10 minutes

>> Chair squats and bicep curls: 12 repetitions

>> Standing leg lift and shoulder raise: 12 repetitions each side

>> Reverse lunge and triceps kickback: 10 repetitions each side

>> Triceps push-up (Figure 13-7) or wide arm push-up (Figure 13-8): 12 repetitions

>> Fold-over glute lift: 12 repetitions each side

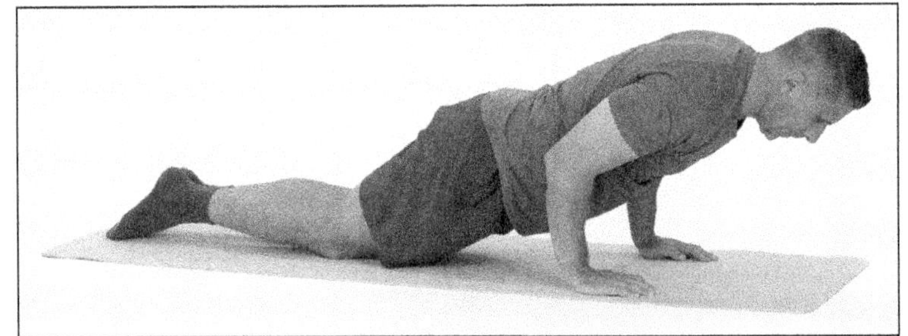

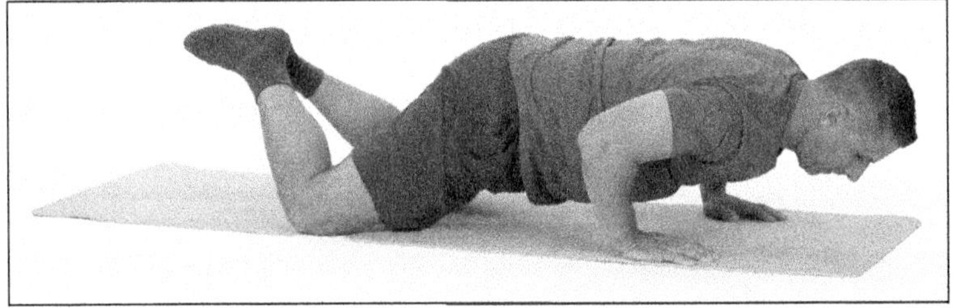

Cardio burst

1 minute

>> Knee Repeaters: 30 seconds each side

Balance

30 seconds

>> Passé hold (Figure 13-9)

Stretch

2 minutes

>> Full-body reach

>> Hamstring stretch

>> Chest opening

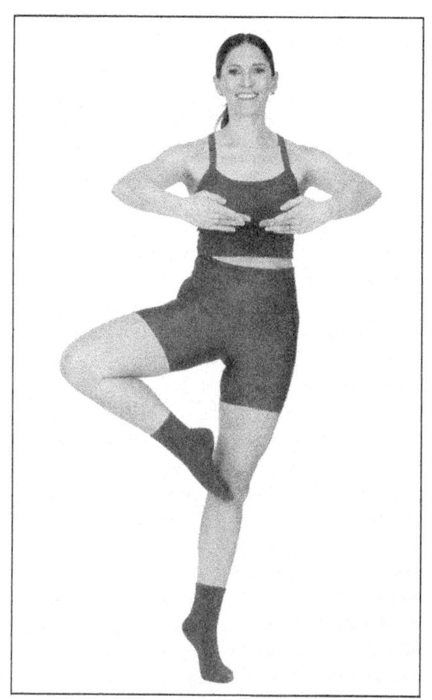

FIGURE 13-9:
A classic passé
hold, with
heel lifted.

Chapter **14**

Movement Snacks

Barre does not have to live inside a workout window or stay on the mat. One of my favorite things about Barre is how easily it fits into real life. What I call "movement snacks" are short, effective exercises you can sprinkle throughout your day, whether you are waiting for coffee to brew, standing at the kitchen counter, taking a break from your desk, or watching TV.

Each movement snack takes less than a minute or two. They are designed to wake up your muscles, reset your posture, and give you a quick burst of strength and focus. The best bit? You do not need special clothing, equipment, or a warm-up. You just need a moment.

Think of these exercises as little reminders to move your body in ways that feel good. Over time, these small moments add up.

Snack-Sized Pliés

This quick plié series is perfect when you are standing in one place for a moment. It gently wakes up your thighs and glutes while helping you feel grounded and upright.

Getting set

Stand tall with your feet in first position or parallel. Lightly hold onto a counter, chair, or desk for balance if needed.

The movement

1. Bend your knees into a shallow plié while keeping your chest lifted.
2. Press through your heels to straighten your legs.
3. Repeat for 10 to 15 slow repetitions.

You can do this while waiting for coffee, brushing your teeth, or standing at the kitchen sink.

Do's and don'ts

» Do keep your knees tracking over your toes.

» Do stay tall through your spine.

» Don't rush the movement.

» Don't drop your chest forward.

Variations

» Add small pulses at the bottom of the plié.

» Hold the plié for 10 counts to increase the challenge.

Snack-Sized Back Attitude

This movement snack targets your glutes and helps you reconnect with your posture, especially after sitting.

Getting set

Stand tall and hold onto a wall, counter, or chair lightly with one hand.

The movement

1. Bend one knee and lift the leg behind you into a small back attitude.
2. Keep your hips square and your torso upright.
3. Lower the leg with control and repeat 10 to 12 times.
4. Switch sides.

This is a great one to do while reading emails, waiting for a meeting to start, or before a long flight.

Do's and don'ts

>> Do keep the lift small and controlled.

>> Do stay lifted through your core.

>> Don't arch your lower back.

>> Don't swing the leg.

Variations

>> Add tiny pulses at the top of the lift.

>> Hold the lift for 10 counts before lowering.

>> Add pulses to the bottom supporting leg.

Snack-Sized Ballet Lunges

These lunges wake up your legs and hips quickly and help counteract long periods of sitting — essential if you spend a lot of time at your desk.

Getting set

Stand near a wall or counter for balance.

The movement

1. Step one leg back into a lunge with your front leg bent ideally at 90 degrees.
2. Bend both knees and press back to standing.
3. Repeat 8 to 10 times, then switch sides.

Try this while waiting for food to heat up or during a quick break at work.

Do's and don'ts

» Do keep your chest lifted.

» Do move slowly and with control.

» Don't let your front knee collapse inward.

» Don't rush through the reps.

Variations

» Add a small pulse at the bottom of the lunge.

» Hold the lunge position for 10 counts.

Snack-Sized Parallel Thighs

This is a classic Barre burner that works quickly, even in tiny doses.

Getting set

Stand with your feet hip-width apart in parallel. Lightly hold onto a counter or chair.

The movement

1. Bend your knees, keeping your chest up and without leaning forward.

2. Hold the position and pulse gently for 15 to 20 counts.

3. Straighten your legs to release.

This one is great while watching television or waiting on a call.

Do's and don'ts

>> Do feel free to raise up onto your heels.

>> Do keep your chest lifted.

>> Don't lock your knees when you stand.

>> Don't hold your breath.

Variations

>> Add baby pulses in your deepest plie.

>> Hold the squat without pulsing for added intensity.

Snack-Sized Battements

These quick leg lifts help improve circulation and wake up your hips and thighs.

Getting set

Stand tall and lightly hold onto a wall or chair.

The movement

1. Lift one leg forward in a small, controlled battement.

2. Lower with control and repeat 10 to 15 times.

3. Switch legs.

This is a great option when you feel stiff after sitting.

Do's and don'ts

» Do keep the movement small and precise.

» Do stay tall through your spine.

» Don't kick your leg.

» Don't lean back.

Variations

» Alternate front and side battements.

» Add a brief hold at the top of the lift.

Snack-Sized Side Lifts

Side lifts target the outer hips and help you feel more stable and upright.

Getting set

Stand sideways to a wall or counter and rest one hand lightly on it.

The movement

1. Lift your outside leg a few inches to the side.

2. Lower your leg with control and repeat 12 to 15 times.

3. Switch sides.

This works well while standing at the counter or waiting for laundry.

Do's and don'ts

>> Do lift from your hip, not your foot.

>> Do keep your torso upright.

>> Don't hike your hip.

>> Don't rush the lift.

Variations

>> Add small pulses at the top.

>> Hold your lifted leg for 10 counts.

Snack-Sized Push-Ups at the Counter, Chair, or Couch

These push-ups strengthen your arms, chest, and core without making you get on the floor.

Getting set

Place your hands on a sturdy counter, couch, or desk. Step your feet back slightly.

The movement

1. Bend your elbows and lower your chest toward your hands.

2. Press back up to straight arms.

3. Repeat 8 to 12 times.

This is a perfect movement during a work break or between chores.

Do's and don'ts

>> Do keep your body in one long line.

>> Do engage your core.

>> Don't drop your hips.

>> Don't hike your shoulders up; keep them relaxed.

Variations

>> Step your feet farther back to increase the challenge.

>> Hold the bottom position briefly before pressing up.

The Part of Tens

Become familiar with the ten most important Barre exercises that build strength and improve posture.

Discover ten ways to upgrade your workout by doing a few key moves well, consistently, and with intention.

Know the right questions to ask when joining a studio, working with a new instructor, or choosing an online class.

Chapter **15**

Ten Important Barre Exercises

arre can look endlessly creative on the surface, but underneath the choreography are a handful of exercises that do the real work. These are the movements I return to in my classes and with my clients, because they deliver results without fuss. Many of these movements also have deep roots in classical ballet and professional dance training, where efficiency, control, and longevity matter far more than flashy tricks. They build strength, improve posture, and help bodies like yours and mine feel more capable in everyday life.

Once these ten exercises become familiar, you will see them showing up in your workouts again and again. They are the steady movements that really give Barre its strength and structure. Think of them as the reliable friends who always show up on time, don't cause drama, and somehow still do all the heavy lifting.

Pliés

Muscles worked: Quadriceps, gluteus muscles, inner thighs, calves, deep core stabilizers

Pliés are the foundation of a Barre workout for a reason. They strengthen the legs while teaching your hips, knees, and ankles to work together properly. From a scientific perspective, pliés improve joint tracking and load distribution, which helps protect your knees over time. In real life, this translates to easier sitting, standing, and stair climbing. And in ballet, pliés are taught on day one because they prepare the body for almost everything that follows. Barre borrows this idea directly. Strong pliés make all other lower-body movements safer and more efficient.

If you ever feel personally victimized by a plié, you are not alone. That just means it's working.

Once you master a good plié, nearly every other lower-body movement becomes more stable and efficient. See Chapter 14 for sneaky ways to add pliés into your day.

Parallel Thigh Work

Muscles worked: Quadriceps, hip flexors, adductors, knee stabilizers

Parallel thigh work is where people new to Barre workouts often underestimate Barre. These small movements create time under tension, meaning your muscles stay engaged longer without needing big, dramatic motion.

Science tells us this is excellent for building endurance and strength. Mentally, it also teaches patience, which your thighs will absolutely test. While ballet often works in turnout, in Barre, we are more likely to work in parallel to build balanced strength and protect the knees.

If your legs start trembling a little, congratulations! You're doing it correctly.

Back Attitude

Muscles worked: Gluteus maximus, gluteus medius, hamstrings, deep core muscles

Back attitude strengthens the glutes without compressing the lower back, which is a big deal. Strong glutes support pelvic stability and reduce strain on the knees and spine. This exercise also quietly improves balance, even if your standing leg feels like it is working overtime.

Attitude is a classical ballet position designed to build hip strength while maintaining lift through the torso. Barre adapts it to focus on stability rather than height or shape. Dancers love it because it is effective, elegant, and endlessly adaptable.

See Chapter 11 for stretches to release tight hips afterward.

Side Leg Lifts

Muscles worked: Gluteus medius, outer hips, pelvic stabilizers

Side leg lifts target the outer hips, which play a major role in balance and knee alignment. Research consistently shows that strengthening these muscles helps prevent common lower-body injuries. In daily life, these muscles help you walk, stand, and stay upright without thinking about it. This movement echoes ballet's emphasis on lateral strength, which helps dancers stay upright, controlled, and injury-resistant during single-leg work.

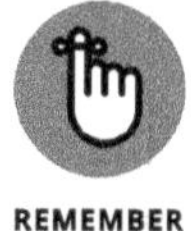

If balance feels tricky here, think of that as information, not failure.

Lunges

Muscles worked: Gluteus muscles, quadriceps, hamstrings, calves, core stabilizers

Lunges are functional strength training. They teach the body how to control weight shifts, something we do constantly in real life. Barre lunges slow things down, emphasizing alignment and control so the nervous system can learn safer movement patterns. Strong lunges mean easier walking, better balance, and fewer awkward moments on stairs.

Relevés

Muscles worked: Calves, ankles, intrinsic foot muscles, lower-leg stabilizers

Relevés strengthen and condition the feet and ankles, which are often overlooked but incredibly important. Studies link lower-leg strength and balance training to improved stability and reduced fall risk as we age. They also demand focus, which is why they feel deceptively challenging.

Relevé comes directly from ballet, where dancers spend years and years training foot strength and control. Barre keeps the essence of that work (without requiring pointe shoes or perfect turnout).

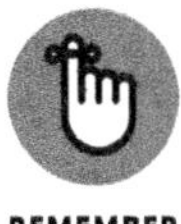

Graceful does not mean easy! Relevés prove this every time.

REMEMBER

Core C-Curve

Muscles worked: Deep abdominals, including the transverse abdominis, spinal stabilizers

The C-curve strengthens the deep core muscles that support your spine. Rather than crunching or gripping, this movement teaches controlled spinal flexion and proper abdominal engagement. Research shows this kind of deep core work improves posture and movement efficiency.

If your neck feels tense, nod slightly forward (think "chin-to-chest") before you move. See Chapter 9 for more support strategies.

TIP

Planks (Modified or Full)

Muscles worked: Deep abdominals, shoulders, upper back, gluteus muscles, stabilizing muscles of the spine — just about all of them!

Planks are one of the most effective — and simple — full-body strength exercises you can do. In Barre, planks are often offered with clear modifications so that you can build strength without strain. You can perform a full plank up on your hands, down on your forearms, and even drop your knees down if you need to.

Holding your body steady against gravity trains deep core muscles and shoulder stabilizers that support posture and protect the spine. This kind of isometric strength work improves endurance and body awareness, and yes, getting stronger in this way really does feel good. While planks are not a traditional ballet step, dancers rely heavily on core stability for balance, transitions, and controlled movement on and off the floor.

Bottom line: Planks help you stand taller, move with control, and get up and down from the floor with confidence. All very **real wins.**

Balance Hold

Muscles worked: Core stabilizers, ankles, feet, hips, postural muscles

Balance work trains coordination between the muscles and the brain. Research shows that balance training improves posture, reaction time, and overall movement confidence. Even short balance holds build awareness and resilience, wobbles included.

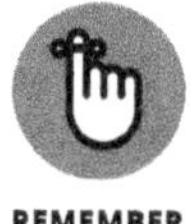

Wobbling a little means you are training, not failing.

Fold-Over Stretch

Muscles stretched: Hamstrings, calves, spinal muscles, lower back

Stretching supports recovery and nervous system regulation, and the fold-over stretch does both. It lengthens the backs of the legs and allows the spine to release tension after strength work. Gentle stretching also helps the body transition out of effort mode.

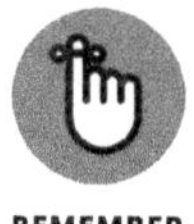

Stretching is not optional. See Chapter 11 for active stretches to add to your routine, and consider setting aside time to do them every day (mornings work for me!).

Chapter **16**

Ten Ways to Supercharge Your Workout

If you have ever finished a workout and thought, "That was fine, but I know it could have felt better," this chapter is for you. After years of teaching classes, training clients, and moving my own body through different seasons of life, I have learned that results do not always come from doing more. They come from doing a few key things well, consistently, and with intention.

These ten strategies are the small upgrades that make a real difference. They are backed by science, shaped by my background as a professional dancer, and tested in my studios and online classes with real people who want to feel strong, capable, and energized without burning out. You do not need to overhaul your routine or add hours to your day. Think of these as simple switches you can flip to help your workouts work harder for you. Try one, try a few, or come back to them whenever things start to feel flat. Small shifts, done often, create big results.

Breathe on Purpose

Breathing sounds obvious, but most people are doing it in a way that makes movement harder than it needs to be. As a dancer, I learned early that breath leads movement, not the other way around, and science backs this up. Deep, belly-based breathing helps regulate your nervous system, improves oxygen delivery to working muscles, and reduces unnecessary tension.

Instead of lifting your chest or shoulders as you inhale, let the breath expand into your belly and rib cage, front and back. Then actually finish the exhale, as if you are gently fogging a mirror. That full exhale naturally engages your core and helps your body stay calm under effort. I always see this in my classes. When clients breathe properly, everything improves. Their balance steadies, their strength feels more accessible, and even challenging moments become manageable.

Warm Up Like You Mean It

A warm-up is not something to rush through or skip when you are short on time. When you warm up with intention, you increase blood flow, improve joint mobility, and prepare your nervous system to respond efficiently. Research consistently shows that even a short, focused warm-up improves performance and reduces injury risk. In my classes, I can always tell who has taken the time to warm-up properly. Their movement looks smoother, their posture is stronger, and they settle into the work more quickly. A five-minute warm-up done well can completely change how the rest of your workout feels, and it's even more important as our body ages.

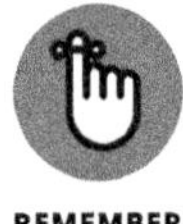

A warm-up isn't just physical, it's mental too. Make your warm-up not just about your body, but also about setting intentions for the workout to come and being present in the movement.

Make Small Moves Count

This is at the heart of my work. Tiny, intentional movements may look modest, but they are incredibly effective. Barre is built on the science of time under focus and tension, which means muscles stay engaged longer, building strength and endurance without impact. I see this surprise clients all the time. A movement may look teeny, then suddenly the muscles are trembling and working deeply. When you focus on precision, alignment, and control, small moves deliver big results. They are efficient, joint-friendly, and sustainable, which is exactly what most bodies need. And the best part? Small moves over time have a big effect.

Train Your Focus, Not Just Your Muscles

Your brain plays a huge role in how your body moves. Studies show focused attention improves motor control and muscle activation. When you are mentally present, your movements are more coordinated and efficient. This is why I cue breath, posture, and intention so consistently in class. You are not just exercising your muscles; you are also training your nervous system to move well. Treat your workout as a focused practice rather than something to rush through, and you will feel the difference immediately, with effects that will only improve over time.

Stop Chasing Perfection

First, the tough news: Perfect form is not always achievable. But here's the really good news: Progress is. When people get stuck trying to do everything perfectly, they often tense up, hold their breath, or stop enjoying the movement altogether. The body learns best through repetition and consistency, not pressure. While I welcome and encourage challenge, I remind my clients all the time that showing up regularly with awareness beats one perfect workout every time. Aim for good form, stay curious, and keep going. Your body adapts when it feels supported.

Use Your Core for Everything

Your core is more than just your abs. It includes deep stabilizing muscles that support your spine and help transfer force through your body. When your core is engaged, your movements become more efficient, and your joints feel more supported. Research shows that core stability improves balance, coordination, and overall strength across the board. In class, I encourage clients to think of the core as the center of every movement, whether they are lifting a leg, reaching an arm, or standing still. When the center is connected, everything else just works better.

Respect Recovery

Recovering well is all part of the work. Muscles rebuild, the nervous system resets, and progress actually happens when you rest. Stretching, gentle movement, hydration, and sleep all play a role. I often tell clients to think about sleep as part of their morning routine rather than just something that happens at night.

Counterintuitive, I know, but how well you sleep directly affects how you move, focus, and feel the next day. I stand for developing simple sleep skills, like consistent bedtimes and winding down properly, which support stronger workouts and better energy overall.

Stack Your Habits with Movement Snacks

One of the easiest ways to stay consistent is to attach movement to something you already do. Behavioral science calls this *habit stacking*, and it works. This is where movement snacks come in. A few pre-matcha pliés while the kettle boils. Side leg lifts while brushing your teeth. A stretch while watching television. I encourage clients to stop waiting for the perfect workout window and start sneaking movement into everyday life. These small moments add up and keep your body feeling engaged and strong throughout the day.

Fuel Simply and Eat Mindfully

Fueling your body does not need to be complicated. What matters most is consistency and awareness. Eating mindfully helps regulate digestion, stabilize energy, and support recovery. One habit I talk about often with my clients is sitting down for breakfast. No screens, no rushing, just 10 minutes to really enjoy your food and eat slowly. Science shows that mindful eating improves digestion and helps your body better recognize fullness and satisfaction. When you start the day grounded and nourished — just for 10 minutes — workouts feel steadier and energy lasts longer.

Finish Strong, Then Let It Go

How you end your workout matters. A calm, intentional finish helps your nervous system transition out of effort and into recovery. Slow breathing, stretching, or a brief balance moment can lower stress hormones and help your body really absorb the work you just did. Then comes the most important part. In the words of Disney's Elsa: *Let it go.*

You do not need to critique or overthink your workout. You showed up, you moved, and that counts. I remind my clients of this constantly. Consistency comes from kindness, so give yourself a moment here.

Chapter **17**

Ten Questions to Ask When Choosing a Class or Instructor

There are a lot of Barre classes out there. Gorgeous, sunlit studios. Slick online platforms. Great playlists that almost convince you this will fix everything. As someone who teaches regularly and works with real clients, I can tell you this: The best class is rarely the flashiest one. It is the one that makes you feel welcome, supported, and capable of coming back again the next week.

I have always tried to foster a sense of warmth and community in my classes, whether you are the chatty, high-energy type or the quiet person who slips in, does the work, and slips out again. Both belong. This chapter is here to help you choose a class that respects your body, your time, and your nervous system, while still being uplifting and motivating.

Do I Feel Welcome Here?

This matters more than the lighting, the mirrors, or how good the playlist is (even though I love a good playlist). A good studio or instructor creates an environment that feels open, relaxed, and human. You should feel comfortable whether you love chatting before class or prefer to arrive, focus, and get moving. You should expect your instructor to be empathic, nonjudgmental, and responsive. A real sense of community does not mean forced friendliness. It just means feeling respected, supported, and at ease from the moment you walk in or press play.

Does the Instructor Explain Things Clearly?

No one enjoys feeling lost five minutes into a class. A strong instructor explains movements clearly and does not assume you already know the choreography, the terminology, or which leg is which. If the class moves so quickly that you spend most of your time guessing, that is not a badge of honor. Clear cues and instructions build confidence and keep bodies safe. That really matters when you're pre- or post-natal, have some limits to your movement, or are a newbie with a learning curve in ahead of you.

Classes that are multilevel — that is, geared to both complete newcomers through to seasoned barre-lovers who seem to have been prima ballerinas in a past life — really win out here.

Are Modifications Offered and Normalized?

For me, this one is non-negotiable. Modifications are what open a class up to almost everyone. Bodies come with histories, limitations, injuries, and off days. A good instructor offers options without making a big deal out of them. Modifying is not failing, it is listening to your body. Instructors who encourage you toward your challenge zone? Great. But classes that treat all bodies the same usually do not serve anyone very well. When teaching new instructors through my Barre brand, Xtend, we program for each body in the room, centering and challenging every student, whether it's their first class or their 1,000th class.

Is There Room for Fun as Well as Fundamentals?

Though instructors should command a respectful room (members should be quiet throughout class and should be discreet if they are entering late or leaving early), workouts can absolutely be fun! Music can be great. You can absolutely enjoy yourself while still respecting alignment, control, and safety. The best classes do both! They make you smile, maybe even laugh, while still doing the work that helps your body feel better in the long run.

Is the Pace Something I Can Grow Into?

The setups should be simple and clear. Cues should reflect how it feels to perform the move, and, when useful, an instructor should offer a demonstration for visual learners. You do not need to keep up with everything immediately. What matters is whether the pace feels achievable over time. Show up consistently, and your strength, coordination, and confidence will increase. A good class allows you to grow into it, rather than making you feel behind from the start.

Does the Class Feel Encouraging Rather than Competitive?

This is the mental side of movement. You should feel encouraged to work alongside others, not distracted by comparison. A good class keeps the focus on your own experience. *Your* body. *Your* effort. *Your* progress. Movement is personal, not a competition with the person next to you who has been doing this for ten years.

Are Warm-Ups and Cooldowns Taken Seriously?

I have said this throughout the book, and I will say it again. Warm-ups and cooldowns matter. They prepare your body to move well and help it recover afterward. If these are consistently rushed or skipped, that is something to notice. Your body deserves a class that respects the beginning and the end, not just the middle.

Does the Instructor Have Experience and Curiosity?

Experience matters. Teaching real people over time builds skill and judgment. At the same time, great instructors stay curious. They continue learning, adapting, and evolving with new research and ideas. You want someone grounded and open, not stuck or showy. Both experience and curiosity matter. This curiosity should extend to you, too: A great instructor will take time to be conscious of any physical and medical conditions, limitations, or injuries you might be working with. Although the onus is on you to speak up, you should feel able to.

Can I See Myself Coming Back?

There is a simple truth in the fitness world that never gets old. The best class is the one you keep going to. If a class fits into your life, feels supportive, and works with your body, that matters far more than chasing the perfect format. Consistency always wins.

How Do I Feel When I Walk Out?

This is the final test. You want to leave feeling taller, stronger, calmer, and quietly proud of yourself. You might feel challenged or tired, but you should also feel better than when you arrived. That feeling is what keeps people coming back, and it is what good teaching is designed to create.

GREEN FLAGS AND RED FLAGS TO WATCH FOR

When choosing a studio to join, a specific instructor to train with, or an online class, the following green and red flags can help you determine whether the fit is right for you.

Green flags:

- You feel welcome right away, even if you are brand new.

- Instructions are clear and easy to follow.

- Modifications are offered without judgment.

- The instructor reminds you to breathe.

- Warm-ups and cool-downs are not skipped.

- You leave feeling worked, supported, and proud of yourself.

Red flags:

- You feel rushed, confused, or invisible.

- Modifications are missing or discouraged.

- The pace feels overwhelming with no guidance.

- The class feels competitive or intimidating.

- Warm-ups or stretches are treated as optional extras.

- You leave feeling tense, deflated, or discouraged.

Index

Numerics

90-degree lifts, 232

10 minutes lower-body sculpt
  chair heel lifts, 234
  chair position, 234
  fold-over glute lift, 235
  knee to elbow crunch, 235
  lunge backs, 235
  second-position pliés, 234
  second-position pulses, 234
  side leg lifts, 235

10 minutes total-body sculpt
  chair squats and bicep curls, 241
  fold-over glute lift, 241, 242
  reverse lunge and triceps kickback, 241
  standing leg lift and shoulder raise, 241
  triceps push-up, 241, 242

10 minutes upper-body sculpt
  90-degree lifts, 232
  arm circles, 232
  balance, 233
  bicep curls, 232
  cardio burst, 233
  genie arms, 232
  stretch, 233
  swimming arms, 232
  temperature arms, 232
  triceps lunge, 232, 233
  V-press, 232

A

abdominal muscles, 18. *See also* core muscles
abdominal stretches, 215, 223, 226. *See also* stretch

abs and torso stretch series, 194–197
Accetta, Matthew, 12
active flexibility drills, 53
active stretching, 187. *See also* stretch
  abs and torso stretch series, 194–197
  balance ending, 204–206
  floor stretch, 200–203
  full-body ballet stretches, 198–200
  seat stretches, 192–194
  upper-body stretch sequence, 188–192
aerobics
  high-intensity and, 13
  moderate-intensity aerobic activity, 14
à la seconde, 62
ankle, 20
  extension at, 52
  flexion at, 51
  stability, 21
anterior pelvic tilt, 24
arabesque, 65–66
arm circles, 100–103, 220, 224, 232
  side, 211
arm crossover, 188, 189, 211, 212
arms
  classical ballet positions
    first position, 43–44
    low fifth and high fifth positions, 46–48
    second position, 45–46
  neutral, 27
  supportive, 32
  swimming and temperature, 108–111
  working, 32
arm sweeps, 232
attitude pose, 63–65
attitude stretch, 193. *See also* stretch

B

back attitude, 108, 145–147, 256–257
  snack-sized, 246–247
back to barre battements, 142–145, 225
balance, 233
  express cardio workout, 240
  express core workout, 238
  express lower-body workout, 235
  express total-body workout, 242
  express upper-body workout, 233
  lower body, 28–29
  mastery with novelty, 40
balance ending, 204–206
  full-body 30-minute workout, 228
  full-body 50-minute workout A, 217–219
  full-body 50-minute workout B, 223
  full-body 50-minute workout C, 226
balance hold, 259
ballet-inspired exercise, 8
ballet lunges, 147–148
  snack-sized, 247–248
ballet movements, 54–62. *See also* port de bras
    ("carriage of the arms")
ballet poses, 63–67
  arabesque, 65–66
  attitude, 63–65
  penché, 66–67
ballet positions
  arms
    first position, 43–44
    low fifth and high fifth positions, 46–48
    second position, 45–46
  feet
    first position, 41–43
    second position, 44–45
ball under lumbar stretch, 195
Barre burn, 28–29
Barre classes or instructors
  challenged or tired feeling, 268
  clear cues and instructions, 266
  consistency, 268

experience and curiosity, 268
focus on your own experience, 267
fun and enjoyment, 267
modifications, 266
questions to ask when choosing, 265–269
sense of community, 266
simple and clear setups, 267
warm-ups and cool-downs, 268
Barre series
  full-body 30-minute workout, 228
  full-body 50-minute workout A, 213
  full-body 50-minute workout B, 220
  full-body 50-minute workout C, 225
Barre shake, 12
Barre workouts, 1, 7–8
  chair, countertop, or wall support, 37
  clothing, 35
  examining main components of, 36–38
  focus, 38
  four pillars (strength, stamina, stretch,
    stability), 10–11
  hair during, 35
  history of, 9–10
  modifications and progressions, 14
  with other forms of exercise, 14
  practicing for a lifetime, 8–9
    low impact, high intensity, 13
    mind–body movement, 12–13
    natural stress-reliever, 13–14
    sustainable strength and mobility, 13
  small moves with big results, 8–9
  in studio or at home, 8
  with walking experienced positive physiological
    effects, 14
battements, 68–69
  back to barre, 142–145, 225
  snack-sized, 249–250
belly-based breathing, 261–262
Berk, Lotte, 9
bicep curls, 90–94, 220, 224, 232
  front, 210
  side, 211

big deep breath, 236
body alignment, 27–28
bottoms up, 182–185, 216, 223
butt, 19

C

cardio burst or series
  express cardio workout, 240
  express lower-body workout, 235
  express upper-body workout, 233
  total-body express workout, 242
carriage of the arms. *See* port de bras ("carriage of
    the arms")
C-curve, 27
  abs, 162–165, 222
  hold, 160–162, 215, 222, 226, 237
  pulses, 237
cervical spine, 17
chair heel lifts, 234
chair position, 234
chair squats and bicep curls, 241
challenge zone, 71–72
chest expansion, 211, 212, 233
  with fold-over, 189, 190
chest opening, 242
classical ballet
  arm position
    first position, 43–44
    low fifth and high fifth positions, 46–48
    second position, 45–46
  feet position
    first position, 41–43
    second position, 44–45
  movements, 54–62
    à la seconde, 62
    derrière, 62
    devant, 62
    développé, 61–62
    passé, 59–61
    plié, 55–56
    port de bras ("carriage of the arms"), 48–49,
      103–104, 125

    relevé, 57–59
    tendu, 56–57
  poses, 63–67
    arabesque, 65–66
    attitude, 63–65
    penché, 66–67
  positions (*see* ballet positions)
classic positions
  back attitude, 145–147
  back to barre battements, 142–145
  ballet lunges, 147–148
  first-position pliés, 124–127
  fold-over series, 155–157
  fourth position, 129–132
  hamstring series, 148–150
  hip circles, 137–139
  parallel pliés, 134–137
  passé press series, 140–142
  resistance band series, 153–155
  second-position cardio, 132–134
  second-position pliés, 127–129
  side lifts, 150–152
closed ribs, 28
clothing, 35
consistency, 38, 264
contraction, 53
cooldown phase, 38
core C-curve, 258. *See also* C-curve
core muscles, 23–24. *See also* abdominal
    muscles; C-curve
  butt, 19
  obliques, 19
  pelvis, 19
    anterior tilt, 24, 25
    control, 24
    neutral, 26
    posterior tilt, 24, 25
  "six pack," 18–19
  strengthening, 37
    C-curve abs, 162–165
    C-curve hold, 160–162
    passé abs, 170–172

core muscles *(continued)*
    plank, 172–174
    scissors, 167–170
    supine lifts, 165–167
  transverse abdominis, 19
core series
  express core workout
    C-curve hold, 237
    C-curve pulses, 237
    crisscross, 237
    plank passé, 237, 238
    scissors, 237
    supine marches, 237
  full-body 30-minute workout, 228
  full-body 50-minute workout A, 215–216
  full-body 50-minute workout B, 222–223
  full-body 50-minute workout C, 226
cross-body stretch, 233. *See also* stretch
curtsy, 70–71
  with side lift, 240
curtsy pliés, 86–87, 224
curtsy triceps, 116–118, 211

D

dance-inspired workouts, 12
deep breath overhead, 233
deep stabilizing muscles, 7, 263
dégagé, 68
demi-plié, 55
depression
  scapular, 18
derrière, 62
devant, 62
développé, 61–62
dynamic movements, 67–71
  battement, 68–69
  curtsy, 70–71
  pivot, 69–70

E

elbow draw-downs, 211
elevation
  shoulder or scapular, 18
equipment, 34
exercise. *See also* warming up
  ballet-inspired, 8
  classic positions
    back attitude, 145–147
    back to barre battements, 142–145
    ballet lunges, 147–148
    first-position pliés, 124–127
    fold-over series, 155–157
    fourth position, 129–132
    hamstring series, 148–150
    hip circles, 137–139
    parallel pliés, 134–137
    passé press series, 140–142
    resistance band series, 153–155
    second-position cardio, 132–134
    second-position pliés, 127–129
    side lifts, 150–152
  lower body, 175–185
    bottoms up, 182–185
    love to hate, 180–182
    side-seat series, 176–180
  upper body
    90-degree lifts, 94–97
    arm circles, 100–103
    bicep curls, 90–94
    curtsy triceps, 116–118
    hinge swing fly series, 115–116
    hug and carriage, 105–108
    port de bras, 103–104
    rowing and puppet, 113–115
    swimming and temperature, 108–111
    triceps lunges, 119–121
    V-press, 111–113
    waltzing, 97–100

express cardio workout, 239–240
  balance, 240
  curtsy with side lift, 240
  jog or march in place, 240
  knee to elbow twist, 240
  march with reach, 239
  parallel squat and arm swing, 240
  second-position plié and reach, 240
  side-to-side lunge reach, 240
  standing knee pulls, 240
  step touch with arm sweep, 239
  stretch, 240
  warm-up, 239
express core workout, 236–239
  balance, 238
  C-curve hold, 237
  C-curve pulses, 237
  crisscross, 237
  mountain climbers, 238
  oblique twists, 237
  plank passé, 237, 238
  plank walkouts, 238
  scissors, 237
  stretch, 238
  supine marches, 237
  warm-up, 237
express workout
  lower-body, 234–236
    balance, 235
    cardio burst, 235
    stretch, 236
    warm-up, 234
  total-body, 240–243
    balance, 242
    cardio burst, 242
    chair squats and bicep curls, 241
    fold-over glute lift, 241, 242
    passé hold, 242, 243
    reverse lunge and triceps kickback, 241
    standing leg lift and shoulder raise, 241
    stretch, 242
    triceps push-up, 241, 242
    warm-up, 241
  upper-body, 231–233
    balance, 233
    optional cardio burst, 233
    stretch, 233
    warm-up, 232
extension, 51–52
  at ankle, 52
  prone, 238, 239
external rotation side stretch, 198–199

F

fascia, 21
feet or foot
  alignment, 20–21
  classical ballet positions
    first position, 41–43
    second position, 44–45
  four points in, 20–21
  pronation, 21
  stability, 21
  stability and alignment, 29
  supination, 21
figure-four stretch, 236. *See also* stretch
first-position lunge back, 81–83
first-position pliés, 124–127
first-position relevé, 213
flexibility, 52–53
flexion, 50–51
  at ankle, 51
floor stretch, 200–203. *See also* stretch
  second-position, 215, 216
floor work, 37
fold-over
  chest expansion with, 189, 190
  second-position, 221, 222
fold-over glute lift, 235, 241, 242
fold-over running/sassy walk, 193

fold-over series, 155–157
  full-body 50-minute workout A, 215
  full-body 50-minute workout B, 221–222
fold-over stretch, 259. *See also* stretch
forward fold with point/flex, 202
fourth position, 129–132
frontal plane, 31
full-body ballet stretches, 198–200. *See also* stretch
full-body 30-minute workout, 227–229
  balance ending, 228
  Barre series, 228
  core series, 228
  stretches, 228
  upper-body series, 228
  warm-up, 227
full-body 50-minute workout A, 209–218
  balance ending, 217–219
  Barre series, 213
  core series, 215–216
  fold-over series, 215
  lower-body floor series, 216
  resistance band series, 214
  stretches, 217–218
  thigh work, 213–214
  upper-body series, 210–213
  warm-up, 210
full-body 50-minute workout B, 218–223
  balance ending, 223
  Barre series, 220
  core series, 222–223
  fold-over series, 221–222
  lower-body floor series, 223
  stretches, 223
  thigh work, 221
  upper-body series, 220
  warm-up, 219
full-body 50-minute workout C, 223–226
  balance ending, 226
  Barre series, 225
  core series, 226
  glute and hip work, 225–226
  lower-body floor series, 226
  stretches, 226
  thigh work, 225
  warm-up, 224
full-body reach, 242
full-out effort, 40

G

genie arms, 232. *See also* arms
glute and hip work, 225–226
green flags, 268–269
grip socks, 35

H

habit stacking, 264
hamstring series, 148–150
hamstring stretch, 194, 236, 240, 242. *See also* stretch
head, 16
high-impact exercise, 13. *See also* exercise
high-intensity and aerobics, 13
hinge swing fly series, 115–116
hip circles, 137–139, 225
  with ball, 213
hip flexor stretch, 214. *See also* stretch
hips
  square off (or box), 28
hug and carriage, 105–108, 220, 224
hyperextend knees, 20

I

intentional movements, 21, 262. *See also* movements
isolation technique, 49–50
isometric exercise, 9, 30. *See also* exercise

K

kinesthesia, 15, 16
knee
  hyperextension, 20
  placement, 29–30
knee-lift march, 234

knee-lift series, 76–78, 210
knee to elbow crunch, 235

L

leg
  side lifts, 235, 257
  supportive, 32
  working, 32
lift with purpose, 31
love to hate, 180–182
lower body, 28–29
  exercises, 175–185
    bottoms up, 182–185
    love to hate, 180–182
    side-seat series, 176–180
  foot stability and alignment, 29
  isometric exercise, 30
  knee placement, 29–30
  static stretch, 31
lower-body express workout, 234–236. *See also* express workout
  balance, 235
  cardio burst, 235
  stretch, 236
  warm-up, 234
lower-body floor series
  full-body 50-minute workout A, 216
  full-body 50-minute workout B, 223
  full-body 50-minute workout C, 226
low-impact exercise, 13, 20
lumbar spine
  for pelvic tilts, 17
lumbar stretch
  ball under, 195
lunge backs, 235
lunges, 257
lying twist, 238

M

march with arm sweep, 241
march with core engagement, 237
march with oppositional arms, 232
march with reach, 239
marking movements, 39–40
mermaid stretch, 196. *See also* stretch
midline, 28
mind–body movement, 12–13
mindful eating, 264
mini pliés, 241. *See also* plié
mini squats, 234
mobility
  sustainable improvement, 13
moderate-intensity aerobic activity, 14
modifications and progressions, 14
motivation, 39
movements
  90-degree lifts, 95–97
  abs and torso stretch series, 195–197
  arm circles, 101–102
  back attitude, 147
  back to barre battements, 143–144
  balance ending, 204–205
  balance mastery with novelty, 40
  ballet lunges, 147–148
  bicep curls, 91–94
  bottoms up, 183–185
  breathe on purpose, 261–262
  C-curve abs, 162–164
  C-curve hold, 160–161
  classical ballet, 54–62
    à la seconde, 62
    derrière, 62
    devant, 62
    développé, 61–62
    passé, 59–61
    plié, 55–56
    relevé, 57–59
    tendu, 56–57
  curtsy pliés, 86–87
  curtsy triceps, 117–118
  dynamic, 67–71
    battement, 68–69

movements *(continued)*
    curtsy, 70–71
    pivot, 69–70
  first-position lunge back, 81–82
  first-position pliés, 125–126
  floor stretch, 200–203
  fold-over series, 156–157
  fourth position, 130–131
  full-body ballet stretches, 198–199
  hamstring series, 149–150
  hinge swing fly series, 115–116
  hip circles, 138–139
  hug and carriage, 106–108
  intentional, 21, 262
  knee-lift series, 76–77
  love to hate, 180–181
  marking, 39–40
  mechanics, 31–32
    lift with purpose, 31
    planes of movement, 31
    range of motion, 31–32
    supportive leg or arm, 32
    working leg or arm, 32
  mind–body, 12–13
  parallel pliés, 135–137
  passé abs, 171
  passé press series, 140–141
  planes of, 31
  plank, 173–174
  plié tendu, 79–80
  port de bras, 104
  resistance band series, 154
  rowing and puppet, 113–114
  scissors, 168–169
  seat stretches, 192–194
  second-position cardio, 132–133
  second-position pliés, 128–129
  side lifts, 151–152
  side reach, 83–85
  side-seat series, 176–179
  supine lifts, 165–166
  swimming and temperature, 109–111
  triceps lunges, 120–121
  upper-body stretch sequence, 188–191
  V-press, 111–112
  waltzing, 98–100
movement snacks, 245
  push-ups at the counter, chair, or couch, 251–252
  snack-sized back attitude, 246–247
  snack-sized ballet lunges, 247–248
  snack-sized battements, 249–250
  snack-sized parallel thighs, 248–249
  snack-sized pliés, 245–246
  snack-sized side lifts, 250–251
  stack your habits with, 264
muscle system, 21

N

natural stress-reliever, 13–14
navel to spine, 26
neck, 16
neutral pelvis, 26
neutral shoulders and arms, 27
neutral spine, 17, 27

O

obliques, 19
open and close series, 210
overhead reach, 240

P

parallel leg stretch, 198. *See also* stretch
parallel pliés, 134–137, 225. *See also* plié
  with ball pulse, 213
parallel thighs
  snack-sized, 248–249
parallel thigh work, 256
passé, 59–61, 108
  parallel, 61
  turned-out, 61
passé abs, 170–172, 223, 226

passé press series, 140–142
pelvic tilts
  anterior, 24, 25
  lumbar spine for, 17
  posterior, 24, 25
pelvis, 19
  control, 24
  neutral, 26
penché, 66–67, 199. *See also* stretch
Pilates, Joseph, 37
pivot, 69–70
planes of movement, 31
plank, 172–174, 211, 223, 226, 258
plié, 55–56, 255–256
  curtsy, 86–87
  first-position, 125–126
  mini, 241
  parallel, 134–137
  on relevé, 213
  second-position, 127–129
  snack-sized, 245–246
  tendu, 78–80, 210, 224
port de bras ("carriage of the arms"), 48–49,
    103–104, 125
positions of ballet. *See* ballet positions
posterior pelvic tilt, 24
posture
  alignment and, 27–28
power
  lower body, 28–29
power center, 24. *See also* core muscles
preparation for Barre first workout
  choosing right equipment, 34
  setting up your space, 33–34
  upgrading your experience with music, 35
  wearing right clothes, 35
pretzel, 193, 226. *See also* stretch
progressions, 14
pronation
  foot, 21
prone extension, 238, 239
prone stretch, 195. *See also* stretch

proprioception, 15, 16
protraction and retraction, 18
puppet, 211
push-ups
  center floor, 211, 225
  at the counter, chair, or couch, 251–252
  triceps, 241, 242

Q

quad stretch, 236, 240. *See also* stretch

R

range of motion, 31–32
rectus abdominis, 18
red flags, 269
relevé, 43, 57–59, 135, 257–258
  first-position, 213
  pliés on, 213
resistance band series, 153–155
  full-body 50-minute workout A, 214
retraction, 18
reverse lunge and triceps kickback, 241
ribs
  closed, 28
rowing, 220
rowing and puppet, 113–115

S

sagittal plane, 31
scapular depression, 18
scapular elevation, 18
scissor crisscross, 215, 223
scissors, 167–170
seated side stretch, 238. *See also* stretch
seat stretches, 192–194, 215, 221, 226. *See
    also* stretch
second-position cardio, 132–134, 213, 225
second-position floor stretch, 215, 216. *See also*
    floor stretch
second-position fold-over, 221, 222
second-position pliés, 127–129, 234. *See also* plié

second-position pulses, 234

second-position stretch, 201. *See also* stretch

shoulder

  and arms, 18

  elevation and depression, 18

  neutral, 27

  protraction and retraction, 18

  square off (or box), 28

shoulder rolls, 232

side leg lifts, 235, 257

side lifts, 150–152

  snack-sized, 250–251

side reach, 83–85, 210, 224

  on floor, 190, 191

side-seat series, 176–180, 216

side-step touch, 234

single-leg stretch. *See also* stretch

  in second position, 201, 202

sit bones, 117

"six pack," 18–19

skeletal muscles, 21

Slick online platforms, 265

spine, 17

  navel to, 26

  neutral, 27

squats

  chair squats and bicep curls, 241

  mini, 234

  parallel squats and arm swing, 240

stability, 11

  ankles, 21

  foot, 21

stamina, 10

standing figure-four, 193

standing fold-over with soft knees, 221, 222

standing leg lift and shoulder raise, 241

standing side bend, 211, 213, 237

static stretch, 31. *See also* stretch

step touch with arm sweep, 239

stop chasing perfection, 263

strength, 10

  lower body, 28–29

  sustainable improvement, 13

strengthen your core, 37, 159

  C-curve abs, 162–165

  C-curve hold, 160–162

  passé abs, 170–172

  plank, 172–174

  scissors, 167–170

  supine lifts, 165–167

stretch, 10–11, 233

  abdominal, 215, 223, 226

  abs and torso stretch series, 194–197

  attitude, 193

  big deep breath, 236

  chest expansion, 233

  chest opening, 242

  cooldown phase, 38

  cross-body, 233

  deep breath overhead, 233

  express cardio workout, 240

  express core workout, 238

  express lower-body workout, 236

  express upper-body workout, 233

  figure-four, 236

  floor, 200–203

  fold-over, 259

  full-body ballet stretches, 198–200

  full-body 30-minute workout, 228

  full-body 50-minute workout A, 217–218

  full-body 50-minute workout B, 223

  full-body 50-minute workout C, 226

  full-body reach, 242

  hamstring, 194, 236, 240, 242

  hip flexor, 214

  lying twist, 238

  mermaid, 196

  overhead reach, 240

  parallel leg, 198

  penché, 66–67, 199

pretzel, 193, 226

prone, 195

prone extension, 238, 239

quad, 236, 240

seat, 192–194, 215, 221, 226

seated side stretch, 238

static, 31

thigh, 214

thigh and hip, 199

total-body express workout, 242

triceps, 189, 233

upper-body (*see* upper-body stretch)

supination

foot, 21

supine lifts, 165–167, 215, 226

supportive limb, 32

sustainable improvement

in strength and mobility, 13

swimming arms, 108–111, 232

swimming series, 211, 225

T

tabletop stretch, 215, 216. *See also* stretch

tabletop twist, 197

technical foundations, 49–53

contraction, 53

extension, 51–52

flexibility, 52–53

flexion, 50–51

isolation technique, 49–50

temperature arms, 108–111, 232

tendu, 56–57

plié, 78–80, 210, 224

thigh and hip stretch, 199

thigh exercises, 221

thigh stretches, 214

thigh work

full-body 50-minute workout A, 213–214

full-body 50-minute workout C, 225

thoracic spine, 17

total-body express workout, 240–243. *See also* express workout

balance, 242

cardio burst, 242

passé hold, 242, 243

stretch, 242

warm-up, 241

transverse abdominis, 19

transverse plane, 31

triceps lunge, 119–121, 211, 220, 225, 232, 233

triceps push-up, 241, 242

triceps stretch, 189, 233. *See also* stretch

tuck position, 24, 25

opposite of, 24, 25

turned-out passé, 61. *See also* passé

U

upper body

90-degree lifts, 94–97

arm circles, 100–103

bicep curls, 90–94

curtsy triceps, 116–118

hinge swing fly series, 115–116

hug and carriage, 105–108

port de bras, 103–104

rowing and puppet, 113–115

starting with, 36–37

swimming and temperature, 108–111

triceps lunges, 119–121

V-press, 111–113

waltzing, 97–100

upper-body express workout, 231–233. *See also* express workout

balance, 233

optional cardio burst, 233

stretch, 233

warm-up, 232

upper-body stretch. *See also* stretch

full-body 30-minute workout, 228

full-body 50-minute workout A, 210–213

upper-body stretch *(continued)*
  full-body 50-minute workout B, 220
  full-body 50-minute workout C, 224–225
  sequence, 188–192 *(see also* stretch)

V

V-press, 111–113, 232

W

waltzing, 97–100, 220
warm-up or warming up, 36, 75, 262
  arm sweeps, 232
  curtsy pliés, 86–87
  express cardio workout, 239
  express core workout, 237
  first-position lunge back, 81–83
  full-body 30-minute workout, 227
  full-body 50-minute workout A, 210
  full-body 50-minute workout B, 219
  full-body 50-minute workout C, 224
  knee-lift march, 234
  knee-lift series, 76–78
  lower-body express workout, 234

march with arm sweep, 241
march with core engagement, 237
march with oppositional arms, 232
march with reach, 239
mini pliés, 241
mini squats, 234
plié tendu, 78–80
shoulder rolls, 232
side reach, 83–85
side-step touch, 234
standing side bends, 237
step touch with arm sweep, 239
total-body express workout, 241
upper-body express workout, 232
working limb, 32
wrist connect, 190, 191

X

Xtend Method, 10, 71

Y

yoga strap series, 203

About the Author

Andrea Leigh Rogers is a wellness entrepreneur, celebrity trainer, and author of the *USA Today* bestseller, *Small Moves, Big Life*. She is the creator of groundbreaking fitness sensation Xtend, a creative combination of Barre, traditional Pilates methods, ballet, and cardio. Featured in *Vogue*, *Harper's Bazaar*, and *Elle*, with live appearances on NBC, ABC, and CNN, she is a popular thought leader in health and movement communities and a youth skincare advocate. Her online workouts have been viewed millions of times.

Her lifelong love of movement started with a dedicated dance practice leading to a career as a professional dancer (most notably as a principal dancer for Walt Disney World Co.), before mastering Pilates as a Comprehensive Classical trainer. Andrea then created her own innovative fusion of core, dance, and Pilates fundamentals, and, encouraged by her clients' response, launched Xtend in 2008 with locations worldwide.

A super trainer on U.S. fitness streaming platform BODi since 2022, Andrea is also a motivational coach and speaker focused on empowering women and girls, building community, and creating movement in all areas of life. She lives in Dallas, Texas, with her two daughters and their dog, Chedi.

Author's Acknowledgments

Thanks to Dan, oh, how I love working with you! Thank you for your partnership, your voice, and your belief in this project. It is what it is because of you.

And Jen, my creative partner in crime, thank you for helping me bring this book to life and for all your insight. I am so grateful for you and your partnership. I couldn't do this without you, Ethel!

Endless thanks to cover photographer Lisa Richov, book interior photographer Sharon Freer, and models Skye Bernardo-Hanson, David Lorber, and Jennifer Cordiner.

A huge thanks to all at Wiley, especially Katharine Dvorak, for her careful stewardship, slick editing, and unfailing enthusiasm. And thanks, as ever, to Todd Shuster and all at Aevitas Creative Management.

Publisher's Acknowledgments

Executive Editor: Tracy Boggier

Senior Managing Editor: Kristie Pyles

Development and Project Editor:
 Katharine Dvorak

Editorial Assistant: Nina Hook

Production Editor: Tamilmani Varadharaj

Cover Image: Courtesy of Lisa Richov,
 Photographer